Biokinetics and Biodynamics of Human Differentiation

Principles and Applications

By

E. BLECHSCHMIDT, M.D.

Professor Emeritus and
Former Director
Anatomical Institute
University of Göttingen
Göttingen, West Germany

and

R. F. GASSER, Ph.D.

Professor
Department of Anatomy
Louisiana State University Medical Center
New Orleans, Louisiana

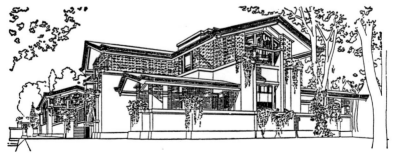

CHARLES C THOMAS • PUBLISHER
Springfield • Illinois • U.S.A.

Published and Distributed Throughout the World by

CHARLES C THOMAS • PUBLISHER

BANNERSTONE HOUSE

301-327 East Lawrence Avenue, Springfield, Illinois, U.S.A.

© *1978, by* CHARLES C THOMAS • PUBLISHER

ISBN 0-398-03654-3

Library of Congress Catalog Card Number: 77-1883

Printed in the United States of America

N-1

Library of Congress Cataloging in Publication Data

Blechschmidt, Erich, 1904-
   Biokinetics and biodynamics of human differentiation.

   (American lecture series; publication no. 1011)
   Bibliography: p.
   Includes index.
   1. Embryology, Human. I. Gasser, Raymond F., joint author. II.
Title.
QM601.B54   612.6'4   77-1883
ISBN 0-398-03654-3

PREFACE

Between 1942 and 1972 serial reconstructions of human embryos were made at the Anatomical Institute of the University of Göttingen. These reconstructions constitute a documentation of the early representative stages of human development and are designated as the "Blechschmidt Collection of Human Embryos." New embryological findings that are based on the reconstructions were published in *The Stages of Human Development Before Birth* (E. Blechschmidt, W. B. Saunders Publishers, 1961), in *Die Pränatalen Organsysteme des Menschen* (E. Blechschmidt, Hippokrates Verlag, 1973) and in *The Beginning of Human Life* (E. Blechschmidt, Springer-Verlag, 1977). A photomicrographic record of the changing position and outer form of the organs in representative stages of human embryonic development recently became available in *Atlas of Human Embryos* (R. F. Gasser, Harper and Row Publishers, 1975). All four of these publications deal solely with *human* development and establish *human* embryology as a field that is completely divorced from phylogenetic considerations and is based entirely on detailed morphological investigations of human material. In this work the new findings from the Blechschmidt Collection will be discussed and explained without reference to any evolutionary considerations. Such an explanation leads to new interpretations of differentiation and development.

Comparisons of isolated data have consistently shown that developmental processes are kinetically related. In other words, developmental movements that occur in one region can be related to the developmental movements occurring at the same time in neighboring regions. As a result of studying such developmental movements it is possible to formulate rules of differentiation. With the application of this knowledge, principles can be derived which generally should be applicable to all living beings. Such principal information is more necessary today than ever before in order to generally interpret the voluminous information that is rapidly becoming available. It should be useful not only to those in the field of medicine but also to those in general biology where new insights into the actions of living matter during development are greatly needed.

A noncontradictory, conclusive and coherent description of the position, outer form and cellular structure of any anlagen (primordium) during development is only possible when changes of the position, shape and structure that take place during development are understood as movements occurring in metabolic fields. In other words, the description of the concurrent development of position (topogenesis), outer form (morphogenesis) and cell structure (tectogenesis) requires a knowledge of the kinetics or movements that occur at each of these levels, i.e. topokinetics, morphokinetics and tectokinetics. Differentiations are discussed from their biodynamic aspect and morphological terms are used because we believe that this approach allows a unique and important entry into the problem of differentiation.

An accurate drawing used in the study of morphology is comparable to the scales used in chemistry in that they are both methods of quantitating and relating things. Kinetic or changing morphology requires a series of drawings of succeeding stages. In other words, accurate illustrations can be interpreted as being states of the movements of the subject which have submicroscopic components. Studies reveal that the movements of organs during development have constructive characteristics and do not contradict the rules of geometry. If a drawing does not conform to the geometric features of an object or contradicts the rules of geometry, it is impossible to point to principles. With this in mind one can make fundamental statements by means of graphic analyses and, in so doing, obtain a clearer understanding of differentiations. We are not implying by this that each developmental process can be reduced to terms and images or be pressed into formulas. We are stating that simple aspects of differentiations such as main direction of growth, areas of relatively slower or faster growth and some submicroscopic movements of materials can even be determined from a purely morphological study.

In this regard, arrows are used in the illustrations to emphasize simple rather than complicated processes. The direction and type of arrows used mean specific things. The more standard ones are: *Outlined arrow* (◁), main direction of growth; *convergent arrows* (▶— ◀), relatively slower growth than that of the surrounding tissue; *divergent arrows with base lines* (◀| |▶), relatively faster growth than that of the surrounding tissue; *tailed arrow* (◀<), submicroscopic movement of materials that become morphologically detectable. All the arrows are valid only if related to a datum point that is in the continuation of the arrow tail. Histochemical and biochemical processes are necessarily immanent in the illustrated features of living tissue. Their investigation requires special techniques and for the present has only just begun. For showing the human embryo in its entirety rather than as a collection of isolated parts, overlabelling of the figures has been avoided.

With the publication in 1911 of *Handbuch der Entwicklungsgeschichte des Menschen* by Keibel and Mall, human embryology began as a field separated from those of botany and zoology. It is no longer sufficient in the field of medicine to base our understanding of human development on comparative embryology. To present human ontogenesis as a deduction from evolution is irrelevant and misleading. In order to describe human development in a clear, nonambiguous way that is completely separate from evolutionary considerations, it has become necessary to use some new terms. Using a new term in many instances is more useful and less confusing than remaining with an old term that has a different connotation. Appropriate terms should be used when the features of human development are unique.   The field of medicine would thereby be relieved of many of the zoological words that are misleading and confusing.   In addition, such new terms should give biologists a better understanding of the facts of human embryology as they are known today.

It was neither the task nor the intention of this book to offer a complete catalogue of data.   We wanted rather to demonstrate by some extremely different examples, that the total field of human embryology should be described under the viewpoint of biodynamic metabolic fields.

E. BLECHSCHMIDT
R. F. GASSER

ACKNOWLEDGEMENTS

THE AUTHORS WISH to express their thanks to Doctor Alphonse Burdi, editor, for the invitation to write a book on the biokinetics and biodynamics of human differentiation for the American Lecture Series in Anatomy. Without his encouragement and support this difficult work would not have been attempted.

The senior author has little command of the English language since his little friends, the embryos, with which he has now been intensely occupied for forty years, have never urged him to learn it. Therefore, he is indebted to his younger coauthor for his personal cooperation, scientific interest and attentive compostion of the English manuscript. The coauthor is grateful to his senior author for the many hours he spent explaining the kinetics and dynamics of differentiations. Without this experience during the coauthor's sabbatical and summer leaves, his participation in this edition would have been an impossible task.

Both authors express their gratitude to Mr. Payne Thomas and his colleagues for the professional and conscientious manner in which they handled the printing and publishing of this book.

E.B.
Göttingen, West Germany
R.G.
New Orleans, Louisiana

ix

INTRODUCTION

$\mathbf{A}$s RECENTLY AS twenty years ago the field of human embryology was incomplete; prior to that time the anatomy of early human embryos was still unknown. In addition, there was much to be learned about the older stages of human embryonic development. Total reconstructions that show the structure of the entire embryo at early stages had not been made. Only the development of organs in isolation was available. Today, human organs are understood as resulting from step by step differentiations of the growing human embryo. From former investigations made by Blechschmidt, it has become known that differentiations are not only the result of a gene effect but are also brought about through growth that is initiated by extragenetic information. Without this extragenetic information the differentiation would not begin. Such a view renews the concept of "development" which should never be even remotely associated with the concept of "evolution."

The principles of differentiation are already evident at the time organs first make their appearance, long before their later development. These principles are the subject matter of this book.

A human ovum cannot be mistaken for an ovum of any other species if the investigations are accurate. Today, there is no doubt that a human ovum, from the moment of its fertilization, contains human chromosomes that are individually specific and cause it, together with the other components of the ovum, to be typically human. There is no longer a question as to whether or not a human ovum will develop into a human being. The question now is *how* do the organs develop from the ovum? In what manner do the outer aspects of the organism change during its distinct development while maintaining its individuality?

In order to answer this question, exact morphological investigations must be carried out. A good deal of information is required before judgement can be made and conclusions reached. It is now apparent that Haeckel's biogenetic law was an erroneous attempt to explain developmental processes. Blechschmidt's human embryological findings that have been gained by accurate investigations have shown Darwin's principles (mutation and selection) as probably being valid for the origin of the species, but they cannot explain the ontogenesis of the organs. The ontogenesis of each individual cannot be derived from phylogenetic facts which have been known since the time of Darwin. This has become clear by recent investigations. Indeed, the findings in comparative anatomy show the relationships of different species but they do not explain the origin of the organs during ontogenetic development. The origin of the species and the origin of the organs are phenomena which fundamentally require different methods of investigation. Anyone using this book must clearly distinguish between the vast field of phylogenetics and the much more exact and understandable field of ontogenetics, particularly the process of differentiation.

Two other points must be understood for the successful use of the information in this book. They are as follows: (1) Hereditary factors are an important, but not the only, condition for the living process of differentiation and (2) genes do not contain any "pattern" of later differentiation. Today, it is known that genes are constants in metabolic processes. Metabolic processes must take place in metabolic fields (Stoffwechselfeld) before genes can function. In the circulatory processes that occur from the cell limiting membrane to the nucleus and back to the cell limiting membrane the genes are points where external stimuli are applied and consequently always have reactive functions. Genes are only a small part of the entire living mass, but because they are constants, they provide for the maintenance preservation of the metabolism. Attention has not been given to this fact previously.

It is common knowledge that all normal cells of the human ovum have the same chromosomes, yet they differentiate in various ways. This fact forces one to conclude that the manner in which genes react must be "dictated" from the outside by local circumstances. The genes themselves do not perform the differentiation process. Besides genetic information there is also extragenetic information that acts from the cell limiting membrane on the cytoplasm. In other words, extragenetic information acts from the outside inwards and in so doing acts on the nucleus. This is why the positional relationship of cells to the neighboring cells is very important for differentiation processes. It is also why differentiation of an organism cannot be attributed exclusively to the genes.

If the pattern for differentiation is not contained in the genes and if differentiation does not occur from the inside, then it must be concluded that the process of differentiation does not begin primarily on the inside but on the outside (outside-inside differeniation). In other words, differentiation is an "external" modification of a given total living organism. In order to establish principles it is very important to understand that the processes of development are spatially ordered movements. Those who cannot accept this will have difficulty accepting the fact that the kinetics of organs that originate from one and the same ovum can be compared. Organs from their very beginning must be compared with each other before rules of differentiation can be established.

Caution should be exercised by those using this book. If one is unaware that life processes are manifested morphologically as momentary spatial images as well as an orderly series of movements and if one is not ready to admit that even chemical reactions have an important physical aspect, then the observations included in this book and the conclusions reached will be of little concern. The knowledge of developmental movements leads to the conclusion that differentiation is an undivided biodynamic process that occurs during development and includes the chemical processes as well. Biomechanical features never occur beside biochemical features, but they always implicate the latter. A biochemical synopsis would be impossible unless one has a fundamental knowledge of the morphology as well as the biokinetics of the organic structures.

It is not the sole intention here to present only the abstract biokinetic principles of differentiation. It is also desirable to point out something of the originality of embryonic human beings. This originality is discernible in many ways; for example, the early human conceptus is master of the whole geometry that it applies to itself. It is never mistaken about any angular sum, and it is never deceived in any surface to volume ratio. It never sets an intersecting point on the wrong site and is master of every physical as well as chemical reaction. Thus, everyone could be enlightened from the abilities of the young embryo, but it is impossible to deduce its originality from scientific findings.

CONTENTS

Page

Preface v

Introduction xi

SECTION I

Early Biodynamic Metabolic Fields

Chapter

1 ONE-CELL HUMAN OVUM 5

2 BLASTOMERIC OVUM AND BLASTOCYST 10

3 ENTOCYST DISC 21

4 AXIAL PROCESS 30

5 THE EARLY EMBRYO 38

6 SOMITES 54

7 LIMITING TISSUES AND INNER TISSUES 68

8 BLOOD VESSELS 80

9 NERVOUS SYSTEM 88

10 HEAD REGION 125

11 TRUNK 137

12 LIMBS 156

SECTION II

Late Metabolic Fields

13 CORROSION FIELDS 183

14 DENSATION FIELDS 187

Chapter		Page
15	CONTUSION FIELDS	194
16	DISTUSION FIELDS	201
17	RETENSION FIELDS	213
18	DILATION FIELDS	228
19	PARATHELIAL LOOSENING FIELDS	244
20	DETRACTION FIELDS	257

Glossary 270
Cited Literature 276
Index 277

Biokinetics and Biodynamics of Human Differentiation

EARLY BIODYNAMIC
METABOLIC FIELDS

At any particular moment during development, an organism functions according to the features its organs have attained at that time. Blechschmidt's investigations support this important concept. There are no organs without functions, either during their developmental period or after they attained a definitive state. This concept also generally applies to the growth functions of each cell and cell aggregations. Consequently, the growth functions of any cell and cell aggregation must be considered in relation to the growth functions of neighboring cells. Neighboring differentiations must be considered during an investigation of the development of any particular cell or cell aggregation (relativity of differentiations). Organs should not be seen as isolated formations but as having associations with the processes of their environment. Human development has not, until now, been studied in this manner.

With this attitude, even early development can be understood as being a functional differentiation which is based to a great extent on very uniform developmental dynamics. This is a basic law of ontogenesis which is formulated as follows: *Ontogenesis occurs by developmental biodynamic differentiations.* These are functional differentiations which generally have developmental dynamic features. They presuppose the life and the idea of a specific

3

human entirety. This statement is very important. If an organism functions according to its characteristics, which change during development, then it follows that the capabilities of a fertilized ovum will be different from those of the blastocyst and implanted ovum. With this in mind, the term "anlage," or primordium, actually means the prerequisites for later developmental processes. It does *not* mean a rigid miniature pattern of the adult organism.

1

ONE-CELL HUMAN OVUM

T HE FIRST DIFFERENTIATIONS are particularly important because they are the beginning of all the following differentiations. It was not until a few years ago that something of the earliest developmental processes of man was known. Some considerations in this field are relevant for orientation.

The fertilized human ovum at the one-cell stage has a characteristic position, a significant outer shape and an extremely complicated inner structure. It is surrounded by a unique basement membrane called the *zona* or *capsula pellucida* which is produced by the follicular epithelium that formerly surrounded it. During the initial period after the follicle cells are lost, the zona makes considerable contact with the molecules composing the uterine tube secretions. The ovum in this positional environment has a spherical shape which is a characteristic feature of its early development. Structurally, the ovum should be thought of as three parts: the exterior, represented by the cell limiting membrane; the interior, represented by the nucleus; and between the exterior and interior a connective cytoplasm that is very active at normal body temperature. The cytoplasm connects the nucleus and the very adaptable cell membrane. This description indicates the idea that all differentiations are necessarily determined by their positional relationship. There is good reason for the as-

5

sumption that every cell represents a field that is called a metabolic field (Stoffwechselfeld). The concept of a metabolic field (cf. 1961, 1977) is very important. It shows that no cell should be thought of as a rigid unity but rather as a momentary aspect of spatially ordered (submicroscopic) metabolic movement (Stoffwechselbewegungen). (These are demonstrated by arrows in the figures.) The same is valid for cell aggregations (tissues), for tissue aggregations (organs) and also for the whole organism at any stage of development. The differentiations could not be described without considering the metabolic field that has been established with fertilization and which is morphologically definable by its cell limits. The continuous transition from developmental stage to developmental stage is based on aligned metabolic movements in metabolic fields.

The concept that the cell is a metabolic field implies for example that the cell limiting membrane cannot act without the nucleus and vice versa, since both are kinetically related to each other by the cytoplasm. With regard to such relationships, the topography of the cell limiting membranes is at present a leading subject of human embryology, the topography of the cytoplasm is a central topic of molecular biology and that of the nuclear structures is the theme of genetics.

It is known that chromosomes are not exhausted in the cell metabolic field. In this manner they are similar to catalysts that are not used up in reactions. They are constants within metabolic fields. Constancy of genetic substances is an important prerequisite for the maintenance of individuality during the process of ontogenesis. The term "genetic effect" is an unfounded abstraction and mainly irrelevant when it is used without regard to the metabolism of the whole organism that begins at the moment of fertilization. The effects of genetic substances should not be compared with "spontaneous instructions" but rather with "replies to instructions." Differentiations arise as functions of the whole organism whether it be one cell or many. In this regard, genetic substances are not a pattern of the later shape of the embryonic or adult organism.

Many examples show morphologically definable features of the active metabolism. Consequently, spatially ordered metabolic movements certainly must occur regularly in metabolic fields during development. In vivo, every cell limiting membrane is part of such a metabolic field, i.e. a field that is related to metabolic processes not only chemically but also kinetically. This shows the particular connections between genetics and morphology which should be investigated.

It is evident that the human ovum consumes oxygen at normal body temperature. There is also no doubt that the oxygen from the exterior reaches the cell limiting membrane before reaching the nucleus. It should be considered that the entering oxygen is not only dissolved, but it also chemically reacts. This means that oxidizable substances move to meet the oxygen entering the cell because of the binding power of oxygen. As a result of these metabolic processes, an unequal surface growth probably occurs in the area of the cell limiting membrane and in the cytoplasm immediately beneath the membrane. This may be the initial event of cleavage.

Usually cleavage is described as being the first cell *"division."* This term, however, is vague since division implies a separation or subdivision. Cleavage is not a division which is a separation, but it is a subdivision resulting in two daughter cells in which process the entirety is maintained. The first subdivision is a process that is stimulated and started externally (by extragenetic stimuli) and is specifically answered internally because of the specific metabolism resulting in differentiations. By means of these differentiations the organism tries to compensate the stimuli and so to maintain its individual metabolism that is given in the moment of fertilization. Numerous investigations up to now have shown that different solid components of the cell regularly contribute to the dynamics of mitosis: the relatively tension-proof cell limiting membrane, the relatively tension-proof spindle-fibers and the liquid between them.

Graphic analysis confirms that during cleavage the surface of the fertilized ovum increases in comparison to its total volume. This enlargement is caused by alterations in the limiting membrane and in the adjacent cytoplasm. Cleavage of the ovum always implies a changing of its proportions: During cleavage the cell always loses its spherical shape (Figs. 1-1 and 1-2), by which process the cell limiting membrane arches unequally. The authors' idea is as follows: The cell limiting membrane is not a

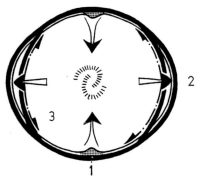

Figure 1-1. Fertilized human ovum with capsula pellucida. Even the one-cell ovum represents a metabolic field with aligned metabolic movements. The outlined arrows (near 2) indicate the changes in shape in the area of the arising poles of the ovum. The tailed arrows (near 1) and the half-headed arrows (near 3) show metabolic movements perpendicular and parallel, respectively, to the cell limiting membrane. The arrows represent an intracellular circuit from the nucleus to the cell limiting membrane and vice versa. Chromosomes are shown diagrammatically in the center.

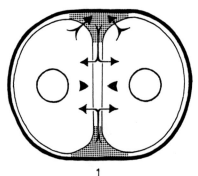

Figure 1-2. Formation movements of the ovum at the end of the first subdivision. The unity of the cell aggregation is preserved by means of the metabolic movements. The tailed arrows show metabolic movements parallel and perpendicular to the cell limiting membrane. The arrowheads represent the reciprocal pressure of the cells to each other which results from metabolic movements.

rigid static structure but is under continuous change, either being built up or being broken down. Regularly, areas of the cell limiting membrane are changed to become substances of the cytoplasm and, vice versa, substances of cytoplasm are incorporated into the limiting membrane. This postulates the existence of an intracellular circuit already functioning within the ovum cell. This circuit represents a rearrangement of submicroscopic molecules which migrate from the limiting membrane towards the nucleus and after having been chemically changed, return to the membrane. This indicates a kinetic order that could not be supposed until now, because the concept of a spatially ordered metabolic field was unknown.

Without the concept of metabolic fields the origin of primary tissues and tissue systems could not be conclusively described at any stage of development. The regular contribution of solid and liquid substances to developmental movements is also valid when primary tissues arise. Growth and differentiation of an early human ovum cannot occur without absorption of materials. Therefore development does not begin from the inside (by genetic information) but externally. The first adaptation of the cells occurs because of the primary growth of the membrane, and thus occurs the first adaption. A developmental stimulus (being extragenetic information) on the cell surface could only effect primarily and then, by means of surface growth, give rise to growth processes in the interior of the cell. All these processes are components of the intracellular cycle mentioned above (such a circuit could also be made evident in plants)[1].

During the intracellular cycle processes the nucleus of the fertilized ovum probably becomes polarized. The polarization of the nucleus seems to bring about the alignment of the equatorial plane and, as a result, the subdivision of the cell body into blastomeres. Even the mitosis shows that the organism remains a living entirety by means of submicroscopic processes, except when real separations of cells give rise to new generations during reproduction.

---

[1]Blechschmidt, E., *Die Lokalisation der antiklinen und periklinen Mitosen* (Naturwiss. Rundschau, 1977).

2

BLASTOMERIC OVUM
AND BLASTOCYST

Despite the fact that most of the physical and chemical data of the first subdivision of the human ovum are unknown, it is apparent that the above changes take place as a result of developmental movements (Entwicklungsbewegungen) with specific main directions. Such movements require energy and therewith are performances with physical work. The blastomeric ovum exhibits the features of such movements.[2]

Since the blastomeric ovum does not notably increase in volume initially, its formation is viewed as a process of internal reorganization. It is reasonable for functional connections to exist between the different parts of the ovum. During formation of the blastomeric ovum, its cells are not only situated beside one another, but they adhere to each other. This is a kinetic principle. The cells can only be separated under notable resistance both in the preserved specimen and in vivo. From the morphological viewpoint, the metabolic field of the early ovum produces an ad-

[2]There is actually no morula stage in human development. This stage has been described for the amphibian and has morphological features which differ from man. The amphibian morula forms neither an amnion nor a chorion. Consequently, the amphibian morula does not show a principle of morphogenesis which could also be valid for human beings.

hesiveness between the cells and draws them together. Connections between these cells are living connections and must not be comprehended as being merely physical. Metabolic processes that expend energy cannot be the same at the surface of the ovum where oxygen enters as they are in the interior. Cyclic metabolic phenomena probably occur not only in the one-cell fertilized ovum, but also in the blastomeric ovum. Examination of a blastomeric ovum suggests that breakdown (dissimilation) products are congested in the interior of the ovum and, after absorbing water, are forced toward the exterior (arrowheads in Fig. 2-1).

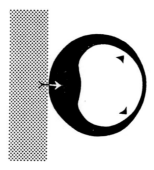

Figure 2-1. Adplantation of the one-chambered ovum (blastocyst) shown diagrammatically. The decidua is stippled, the wall of the blastocyst is black; the intercellular substance is white. The thick-walled segment of the blastocyst is referred to as the ovum disc. The tailed arrow represents the movement of the nutrients; arrowheads indicate fluid pressure.

It is apparent from morphological observations that during extreme cell diminution, liquid collects in the internal part of the ovum forming the first intercellular substance; this process gives rise to the *blastocyst*. The liquid is mainly derived from the cells. Since the cells do not multiply synchronously, the intercellular substance forms at different rates. This causes an eccentric cavity to form in the ovum rather than a central symmetrical one. With this, polarity of the ovum becomes noticeable. The blastomeres push themselves apart eccentrically by the production of the intercellular substance. Peripherally the cells remain adherent to one another by an attraction between their adjacent membranes causing a firm connection. All cells of the blastocyst have a shape that corresponds to their position; the shapes differ according to their adaption to their position. In a cell aggregation, no cell has been detected to have a shape according to some inherent cellular phenomenon such as would be necessary in an artificially constructed mosaic.

Before implantation begins, the blastocyst liquid becomes more eccentric in its position. Where the wall of the blastocyst is extremely thick the outer surface area appears to remain small. Even by the fourth day of development the total volume of the blastocyst does not detectably change compared to that of the one-day ovum. At that time, the approximately 100-minute blastomeres are so diminished that their total volume (composing the wall of the ovum) is less than half the total volume of the ovum (wall plus liquid contents) (Fig. 2-1). This observation is of interest because it demonstrates that the release of substances from the cells is a way of differentiation. In other words, the transport of materials within the metabolic field (Stoffwechselfeld) of the blastocyst are also metabolic movements (Stoffwechselbewegungen) that are spatially ordered. The coagulation capability of the blastocoel liquid leads to the conclusion that the liquid has an osmolarity that, from its beginning, is functionally important for the maintenance of the blastocyst shape. This interpretation is the only way the thick-walled and thin-walled segments of the blastocyst can functionally be explained. The cells in the thin-walled segment are probably less resistant to the osmotic pressure of the blastocoel liquid, causing them to flatten because of the pressure. This means that the blastocyst, with its thicker (discal) and thinner (antidiscal) wall segments, not only has a polarized shape but is functionally polarized as well. This is important since it is known that the blastocyst normally attaches to the uterine mucosa only at its discal pole.

Adplantation and implantation also demonstrate an effect of spatially ordered metabolic movements. Such movements are living processes. The attraction that the blastocyst has for the uterine mucosa may be more of a function of the blastocyst than of the uterine mucosa (Fig. 2-1). In other words, the blastocyst may be able to draw itself to the mucosa. This process is a pre-liminary and very original suckling function. Noting that, it should be emphasized that a very early developmental process is comparable in functions with a later one. The osmolarity that is characteristic of the blastocoel fluid would be necessary not only for the stability of the blastocyst wall but also for the process of implantation. It would be a prerequisite for further development. Polarization of the blastocyst is an example of contrasting differentiation. Such differentiations will be seen again and again during the later stages of development.

With the beginning of implantation the ovum receives a new positional relationship and assumes a new shape that corresponds to its new position. Since the structure of the implanted ovum is necessarily related to its position and shape, that also changes. It is a consistent observation that *position, shape and structure are kinetically related throughout development.* It is so consistent as to be a rule. Actually, the events of development are processes that take place at different orders of magnitude and are always kinetically related.

During the gradual increase in size of the ovum and its disc, growth of the outer and inner sides of the disc is probably due to the supply of nutrients from outside the cell as well as from the blastocoel. It is most likely that the cells of the thin-walled part of the blastocyst release substances into the blastocoel, while the wall extends and its cells flatten. As a result of the absorption of nutri-ents, the ovum (blastocyst) disc protrudes into the cavity of the ovum (blastocoel) (Fig. 2-2, near *1*). The thickening of the inner portion of the disc gives rise to a second cavity. Some cells probably perish inside the disc causing a zone of high osmolarity that is the anlage of the dorsal entoblast chamber (amniotic cavity, Fig. 2-3, *2*). Fluid from the adjacent cells flows into the anlage of the dorsal entoblast chamber. Due to this flow these cells become polarized, i.e. they become epithelial. Epithelial cells always ab-sorb nutrients from one side and deliver katabolites at the other. As a consequence, they are able to expand in surface area.

Thus, at the beginning of the second week, two cysts (liquid plus wall) have developed which are closely connected and form a

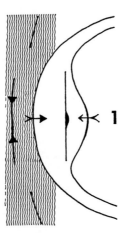

Figure 2-2. Diagram of the implantation area of the blastocyst (approximately 5 days). Convergent arrows show the principal alignment of the cells in the basal decidua. Tailed arrows indicate supplying metabolic movements. The small black area between the tailed arrows represents the arising dorsal entoblast chamber (anlage of the amniotic cavity). *1*, blastocoel

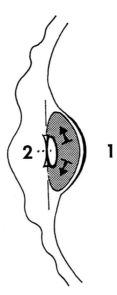

Figure 2-3. Diagram of the thick-walled part of the blastocyst at the end of the first week. Convergent arrowheads show the restraining function of the amniotic anlage. Divergent arrows with base lines represent growth of the ectoderm. *1*, blastocoel; *2*, dorsal entoblast chamber.

disc between the two liquid foci (the primarily developed ventral blastem fluid and the secondary arising dorsal blastem fluid). The whole group of cysts is called the entoblast, the disc is the entocyst disc of the entoblast.

The cell aggregation of the entocyst disc is relatively thick (coarse plus dense stipple in Fig. 2-4) whereas the other epithelial walls of the cysts are relatively thin (dotted broken line and thick line between the convergent arrowheads in Fig. 2-4). From sections it may be seen that the thickening of the entocyst disc is regularly related with the thinning of the rest of the walls of the two cysts (amnion and yolk sac wall). Apparently here an interior rearrangement once more occurs (separating of components). There is a good reason for the conclusion that the nutrients are

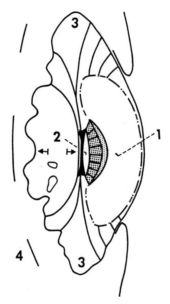

Figure 2-4. The seven day two-chambered ovum during implantation, showing the main alignments of the cell limiting membranes. *1*, ventral blastem fluid in the former blastocoel; *2*, doral blastem fluid in the dorsal entoblast chamber; *3*, equator of the ovum; *4*, basal decidua. Divergent arrows with base lines represent the thickening growth of the ectoblast establishing the trophoblast. Convergent arrowheads show the restraining function of the amnion anlage. Ectoderm is the densely stippled area, endoderm is the coarsely stippled area.

delivered from the flattened cells. Those substances diffuse through the blastem fluid into the disc. It is probably not accidental that the relatively thick entocyst disc arises between the early yolk sac fluid and amniotic fluid.

With the formation of the dorsal entoblast chamber, the cell aggregation between the fluid in this chamber and that in the blastocoel becomes bent concavely towards the amniotic cavity. This cell aggregation is compressed more and more on its concave side. It therefore becomes bilaminar at the beginning of the second week of development. The thicker layer adjacent to the dorsal entoblast chamber is the ectoderm. The thinner layer adjacent to the blastocoel is the endoderm. These two layers constitute the entocyst disc (Figs. 2-3 and 2-4).

By diminution of its cells the early amnion is retarded in growth and stretched. This causes the amnion to exhibit a local resistance against the growth of the entocyst disc and to appear as a restraining apparatus (convergent arrowheads in Figs. 2-3 and 2-4). Liquid gradually accumulating in the dorsal entoblast chamber is referred to as the dorsal blastem fluid. It can be contrasted with the ventral blastem fluid which is the former blastocoel fluid. The terms "dorsal" and "ventral" refer to the layers of the entocyst disc between the two liquids.

From what has been said, the establishment of the topographic and histologic features of the bilaminar stage of human development are understandable in kinetic terms. This differentiation is a necessary prerequisite for the occurrence of all subsequent differentiations. A basement membrane that usually forms under thick epithelium develops in the zone between the two blastoderms of different thicknesses (ectoderm and endoderm). The basement membrane is adherent to the ectoderm. After formation of the basement membrane, the two layers appear as *limiting tissues* (Grenzgewebe) with contrasting characteristics. The ectoderm is thick while the endoderm is thin. The two layers are connected by the basement membrane. Each layer has one border that is firm (basement membrane) and one border that is liquid (respective blastem fluid). Cells in such a position (between two media of different firmnesses) are characteristic of epithelia. In regard to the position of limiting tissues, they should not be thought of as epithelia that are only coverings which function to unilaterally protect the stroma. The term limiting tissue should be used as an extension of the term epithelium. Limiting tissue (usually called epithelial tissue) stresses the fact that it consistently has two different media adjacent to it; one is liquid, the other is relatively firmer and is called stroma. As will be shown later, very orderly metabolic movements occur in the stroma.

In accordance with the concept of limiting tissues, not only cell aggregations are important in the stepwise process of differentiation, but the collections of liquid are also very significant. In the second week both the collections of cells and liquid together exhibit the fact that already the early anlagen are a functional system. As was stated previously, the collections of liquid and their immediate enclosing limiting tissues are referred to as the dorsal (amniotic cavity) and ventral (yolk-sac cavity) entoblast chambers. A secondary yolk sac that is observed in other primates is nonexistent in human beings. At the beginning of the second week, both chambers are enclosed by the outer part of the early ovum called the *ectoblast*. Together the two chambers form the epithelial anlage of the inner part of the ovum referred to as the *entoblast*. As mentioned above, the outer layer of the ovum where its wall is thick attracts or draws itself to the superficial part of the decidua (implantation). Penetration of the decidua is the result of very intense metabolism which gives rise to a metabolic field that is congested with products from both the decidua (maternal) and the blastocyst. In the area of this metabolic field, maternal cells are destroyed with the release of substances that provide the ovum with nutrients (exotrophe). The term *exotrophe* is used to indicate that at the beginning of the second week, nutrients for the ovum are produced at its periphery through specific metabolic processes. These nutrients are used for further development of the ovum. Therefore, it can be stated that positional relationship also plays an important role in the transport of submicroscopic substances.

With implantation the mass of the ovum increases mainly near its implantation pole where it is in intimate contact with the decidua. This is another example of metabolic movements that take place with a specific spatial arrangement (spatially ordered metabolic movements). The ectoblast at the implantation pole is particularly thick and can now be properly referred to in a functional term as the trophoblast, because it extensively serves for the nutrition of the blastocyst. The antidiscal wall of the blastocyst remains thin for several more days (thin part of the ectoblast) (Fig. 2-4). Not until about the twelfth day is the entire ovum implanted and surrounded by the uterine mucosa which then covers over the antidiscal pole. The surface area and thickness of the ovum increase primarily in the region where it is in contact with nutrients, i.e. near the discal pole. Due to the position of the ovum on a large source of nutrients, it becomes lens-shaped. As the position and shape of the ovum change, the main growth occurs in the region of its equator. The equator zone becomes particularly cellular. Here, the curvature of the ovum becomes greatest and its contact with the source of nutrients is largest. Corresponding with the mentioned topokinesis, absorption of nutrients is easiest and surface growth is most accelerated in the equator zone.

The undulating relief formations and the lacunae are mainly in the thick part of the ectoblast (fetal part of the arising placenta) (Fig. 2-4). They are indications of an intensive surface growth. Positive relief formations are morphological signs of locally increasing surface growth and thickness. However, negative relief formations are signs of retarded growth. Positive reliefs allow the formation of villi which occur in the third week of development. Breakdown products collect between the villi, giving rise to the lacunae. The paths of the maternal part of placental circulation develop as a confluence of the lacunar contents. The direction of the paths of the communicating ectoblast lacunae verifies the location of metabolic gradients, i.e. spatially ordered metabolic movements. Such metabolic movements are very distinct near the end of the second week. A principle of developmental dynamics is revealed here, viz, *collections of liquid intercellular substances with a sufficiently strong metabolic gradient lay the ground work for vessel formation.* Also, in later development the vacuolization of tissue in a metabolic field precedes vessel formation.

The multicellular ovum contains a large quantity of water and is distended. Its semiliquid intracellular contents, together with its intercellular liquids, exert fluid pressures and are functioning components of the distended ovum as a whole. If the entire ovum is considered as a static structure, during development the distribution of the liquid products along with the membrane systems would show the ovum to be built as a trajectorial structure (Fig. 2-4). "Trajectorial" means that directions of the structures are mainly parallel and perpendicular to the outer surface of the whole system. These aligned structures represent the main directions of tension in aggregations of living cells. Materials in the ovum are transported primarily according to the trajectorials. Disorderly diffusion material is not evident in any orderly structural medium. This means that in the stage shown in Figure 2-4, molecules are transported from the equator to the entocyst disc and along the basement membrane of the ectoderm and are then taken up by the cells vertical to the basement membrane. Without an orderly distribution of the biomechanical tensions, it would be impossible to understand the manner in which the metabolism of the ovum retains its particular shape.

The trajectorial structure, which is demonstrated by way of drawings, shows that during early development the metabolism of the cells manifests itself by constructive forming stresses (Gestaltungskräfte). In other words, the trajectorial structures show the constructive formative function of the ovum as a fundamental feature for its metabolism. In the stage shown in Figure 2-4 the thick epithelial layer (anlage of the outer germ layer or ectoderm) is an example of a trajectorial formation that is very orderly. The cells here are arranged perpendicular to the basement membrane at one end and perpendicular to the surface at the other. The main directions of the trajectorials can be understood as signs of particularly simple relationships between the shape and structure of the young tissue independently of whatever biochemical and biophysical data will be found in the future.

If the dorsal blastem fluid (anlage of the later amniotic fluid) determined the shape of the ectoderm because of its relatively higher pressure, the ectodermal cells would then be oriented tangential to the amniotic space and become flat. This, however, is not the case. To the contrary, the ectodermal cells are oriented vertical to their basement membrane and also vertical to their free surface. Because of this arrangement, each cell probably exerts during growth a counter pressure against adjacent ectodermal cells. In contrast to this, the amnion regularly shows flattening both as a whole and with its individual cells. The developmental dynamics of these formations is that the amnion behaves in vivo as a layer that is resistant to growth of the entocyst disc *(see* convergent arrows in Figs. 2-3 and 2-4). The growth resistance of the amnion gives it a passive role in regard to its formative functions. Because of the growth resistance of the amnion, the ectoderm and adjacent thin endoderm protrude convexly in the direction of least resistance, toward the blastocoel. Thus, the ectoderm and the young amnion appear to share the formative work of the embryonic anlage, but in different ways.

The more the vault of the young ectoderm becomes visible the closer the newly produced cells press together at the concave side of the vault and the more numerous become the intercellular gaps per unit area. The intense surface growth of the ectoderm (Fig. 2-3, divergent arrows) is accompanied by an increased quantity of the adjacent dorsal blastem fluid. Accordingly, it could be discussed whether the ectoderm releases fluid into the early amniotic space as it begins to vault and move away from the young amnion. Such a movement could cause fluid to be drawn into the early amniotic space because of pressure differences. This is caused especially by perished ectodermal cells which lie in the amniotic cavity and exert an osmotic pressure. Observable evidence for this assumption is still lacking. In the second week of development, the volume of the early amniotic space increases rapidly. There is nothing to support the theory that the dorsal blastem fluid is a metabolic product of the amnion, that is, an "amniotic fluid" in the strict sense. It is unreasonable to consider the thin amnion as the source of the amniotic fluid. In the later stages of human development, the amnion is almost devoid of vessels.

3

ENTOCYST DISC

No one has previously attempted to describe the differentiation of the ovum during the second and third weeks as movements. This shall be done by determining what developmental movements can be demonstrated as changes in position, shape and structure of the implanted ovum.

At the end of the second week various layers of the ectoblast become established as the mass of the ovum increases. These differentiations result from the differential surface growth of the cell aggregations. The relationships of position, shape and structure of these layers lead one to believe that these cells are immediately related biodynamically. The spatial features of differentiation are manifestations of these relationships.

Principally, the membrane systems are apparently closed microscopically but submicroscopically they are open. If this be the case, then molecular as well as submolecular particles could migrate in vivo from cell to cell and from tissue to tissue. The ovum enlarges quickly at its surface by appositional growth because of the assimilation of nutrients from the outside. As this occurs, more and more of the tissue in the transitional region between the ectoblast and the entoblast becomes reticular in appearance (Fig. 3-1, 3). The cells in this zone become flat and small. This change in shape indicates that the cells lose some of their contents.

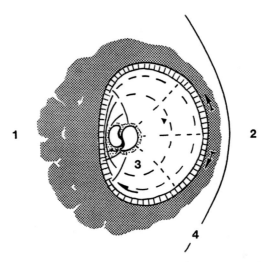

Figure 3-1. A recently implanted two-chambered ovum. *1,* site of basal de-cidua; *2,* site of uterine cavity; *3,* anlage of the chorionic (mesoblast) cavity. Interrupted lines show the principal alignments of the cell limiting mem-branes of expanding mesoblast. Divergent arrows show the surface growth of the ectoblast. Fluid pressure of the preventral blastem fluid in the develop-ing chorionic cavity is shown with arrowhead. Tailed as well as half-headed arrows indicate parmeation-type metabolic movements.

The lost material becomes intercellular substance between the cells. This first inner tissue of the ovum is referred to as the mesoblast, and its appearance is characterized by the accumulation of intercellular substance. The intercellular substance fills the in-terstices which enlarge as the intercellular substance increases. Even though the mesoblast is very delicate and loose between the ectoblast and the entoblast, it appears to be very resistant to the tensions in the surrounding epithelia to which it is in contact. It not only connects the ectoblast and entoblast spatially but also bio-dynamically. Its tissue meshes guide metabolic products from the ectoblast to the entoblast along the limiting tissues. A network of capillaries is evident for such metabolic movements at the begin-ning of the third week.

In subsequent chapters it will be seen that the *limiting tissues* (Grenzgewebe) are structurally characterized as being very cellular with almost no intercellular substance. On the other hand, *inner tissues* (Binnengewebe) have large quantities of intercellular substance. Accordingly, limiting tissues and inner tissues grow in surface area and in volume, respectively. By comparing one developing region with another, a consistent fact becomes evident, viz, when tissue becomes stretched in three dimensions, e.g. mesoblast, the volume of its cells is reduced with the release of intercellular materials into the interstices. From observations, it may be concluded that mesoblast formation, from the kinetic viewpoint, results from the unequal growth rate of the ectoblast and entoblast. This concept is supported by the observation that cells of the inner portion of the mesoblast initially become septal-shaped, then trabecular and finally become so thin that they rupture, thereby forming the cell-free mesoblast (chorionic) cavity. The mesoblast cavity (anlage of the chorionic cavity) would therefore be a dehiscent zone between the ectoblast and the entoblast, which have different surface growth rates (Figs. 3-1 and 3-2). Experiments on various specimens have shown that cells of the mesoblast become attracted by the neighboring epithelia but are repelled from each other by the fluid pressure of the intercellular substances.

As a result of the inner tissue of the ovum rupturing, the chorionic mesoblast gradually becomes the lining of the ectoblast (Wandmesoblast) as it rapidly increases in circumference while the entoblast becomes encapsulated by a covering layer of mesoblast cells (covering mesoblast, Hüllmesoblast, Fig. 3-2). The two-chambered entoblast together with its covering mesoblast is referred to as the *entocyst*. Together with its bilaminar *entocyst disc*, which is situated between dorsal and ventral blastem fluids, it is not only a formal but also a biodynamical unity. The term entocyst disc refers to the position of the disc in the entocyst which is very important for its further development. Here again, position, shape and structure are closely interrelated.

The mesoblast covering the two-chambered entoblast becomes relatively thick in the region of the yolk-sac wall while only a thin layer of mesoblast cells is evident in the region of the amnion and chorion. The following observation leads to a biodynamic interpre-

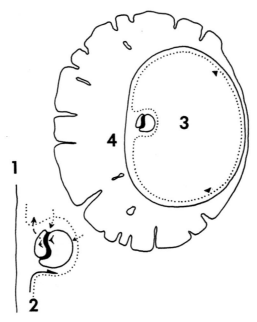

Figure 3-2. A three-chambered ovum. The entocyst contains the dorsal (amniotic) and ventral (yolk sac) chambers filled with dorsal and ventral blastem fluid. *1*, black line representing the cytotrophoblast; *3*, chorionic cavity
filled with preventral blastem fluid; *4*, thick portion of ectoblast (trophoblast). The dotted line (*2*) shows the border between mesoblast and chorionic cavity. To the right of *4* the body stalk joins the chorionic mesoblast
(Wandmesoblast) and the mesoblast which covers the entoblast (covering
mesoblast = Hüllmesoblast). Arrowheads represent fluid pressure of the chorionic fluid. In the inset drawing (lower left), the dotted arrows indicate
infiltration, the half-headed arrow shows parmeation and the tailed arrow
indicates permeation.

tation of the described facts. The nuclei of the yolk-sac mesoblast
cells are large and loosely structured, whereas those of the amniotic
mesoblast cells are small and dense. This indicates that water
balance is of considerable importance in the various local differentiations.

At the end of the third week, the mesoblast cells covering the
yolk sac are mainly aligned perpendicular to the yolk-sac endoderm. They multiply rapidly and become closely packed, with

their cell body and nucleus adjacent to the chorionic cavity. The very thin processes of the cell bodies that are surrounded by liquid intercellular substance attach to the yolk-sac endoderm. This arrangement can be seen easily in the early umbilical region of human embryos approximately 3 mm in length. The yolk-sac wall is known to be under tension. In this system, the living cells of the yolk sac exert biodynamic pressure stresses against one another.

From the regularity of the structure it is again evident that metabolic movements are directed. The alignment of the cell limiting membranes of the covering mesoblast is understandable as a momentary view of spatially ordered metabolic movements. The alignment indicates a polarization of the cells. The tiny contacts between the covering mesoblast cells and the yolk-sac endoderm are probably beneficial in the metabolism of yolk-sac endoderm and, as a result, nourish the entocyst disc. In support of this is the fact that the peripheral part of the circulation, i.e., chorionic blood vessels, are not yet present when the entocyst disc first appears. There are as yet no vessels in which the blood could transport nutrients and katabolites along the yolk-sac endoderm. The amniotic mesoblast is extremely thin and is composed of flattened cells that cover the thin amniotic epithelium. Because of this morphology, it would be impossible for the amnion to develop an important source of nutrients for the entocyst disc. Some endotrophe from the flattening chorionic cells is probably guided to the entocyst disc along the tangentially straightened amniotic cells and is then distributed by way of the basement membrane of the ectoderm. The intercellular substances in the early inner tissue (mesoblast) do not stagnate but flow along the neighboring limiting tissue. This metabolic movement is called a parmeation. The parmeation of intercellular substances in the prime inner tissue is important for giving rise to the vascular circulation. The blood flow along the neighboring epithelia is also a parmeation. The different metabolic movements *(along, and through limiting tissue* and *into* inner tissue equals *parmeation, permeation* and *infiltration,* respectively) are shown in Figure 3-2 by arrows. The eleven-day blastocyst (Carnegie no. 7699)[3] and the twelve-day blastocyst (Carnegie no. 7700)[4] support this assumption.

The mesoblast cells at the periphery of the expanding chorionic cavity and at the vortex of the amnion are stretched in two dimensions whereas the yolk-sac mesoblast is composed of thick cells. The two different cell shapes could be a result of the fact that the circumference of the yolk sac does not increase as fast as the circumference of the ectoblast. As a result, the covering mesoblast cells of the yolk sac remain close together since their growth rate is equally distributed. The shape and structure of the yolk-sac wall leads to the conclusion that the biomechanical tension in the wall is supported mainly by the growing cells of the covering mesoblast rather than by the pressure of the yolk-sac fluid. In any case, in the third week the covering mesoblast of the yolk sac has thickened in relation to the yolk-sac endoderm. The thickening is the result of a high cell-division rate in conjunction with a large accumulation of intercellular fluid.

There is support for the concept that substances are transported perpendicularly through the surface of the yolk sac. These metabolic movements presuppose a metabolic gradient which is directed towards the yolk sac endoderm. Obviously, this gradient results from growth of the entocyst disc. The well-known blood islands show that the yolk sac contributes to the distribution of nutrients for the early embryo.

At the beginning of the third week the intercellular fluids merge in the mesoblast covering the yolk sac. As a result, space is available for the intense vacuolation that initiates the formation of the first blood islands with afferent and efferent pathways in the early embryo. With the appearance of the yolk-sac vessels at the end of the third week, the initial main path of metabolic movements (perpendicularly through the yolk-sac wall) is gradually replaced by the metabolic movements of the vascular system. The vascular system transports nutrients parallel (parathelial) to the endoderm. From this, it becomes obvious that biomechanical

---

[3]Hertig, A.T. and Rock, J.: Two human ova of the previllous stage, having an ovulation age of about eleven and twelve days, respectively. *Carnegie Contr. Embryol., 29:*127, 1941.
[4]*ibid.*

tensions, as well as metabolic movements, exhibit directions that are perpendicular to one another. Main directions of tension should not be limited to expressions of only static features. They also may signify the main directions of metabolic movements, i.e. assimilations and dissimilations. It is reasonable for even the very narrow interstices between cell-limiting membranes to be functional. Material movements directed perpendicular to each other are also important processes in the area of a single cell. Additional support for this concept will be forthcoming. Permeations and parmeations (para-) refer to metabolic movements through membranes and parallel to membranes, respectively (Fig. 3-3).

In summary, the difference in kinetics of the early amnion and the early yolk sac is as follows. The dorsal entoblast chamber grows with the help of the blastem fluid that accumulates within

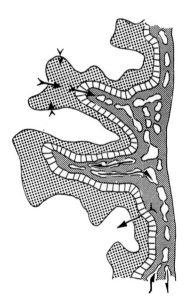

Figure 3-3. The main directions of metabolic movements are shown in chorionic villi of the ovum presented in Fig. 3-2. The tailed arrows illustrate permeation in the limiting tissue and the half-headed arrows show parmeation in the stroma. The epithelium is coarsely stippled and the vacuolized stroma is densely stippled. The cytotrophoblast is hatched.

the chamber. The pressure of the accumulating fluid is accompanied by a noticeable stretching of the amnion, particularly in the area of the vortex. As a result, the amnion becomes thinner as it enlarges with the chamber. The mesoblast cells covering the amnion are aligned tangential to the surface of the chamber. This arrangement is a sign of increasing fluid pressure. In contrast to this, the wall of the ventral entoblast chamber thickens. Here, the covering mesoblast cells are aligned perpendicular to the chamber. This is a manifestation of the biomechanical pressure from the mesoblast cells in this area, which are multiplying and enlarging perpendicularly to the adjacent limiting tissue.

What growth functional significance could the dorsal entoblast chamber, and particularly the amnion, have on the early shape of the ovum? The morphological changes can be interpreted in the following way. When the entocyst disc first appears, it protrudes into the ventral blastem fluid, yielding to the growth resistance of the amnion (Fig. 2-3). As soon as the volume of the dorsal entoblast chamber has enlarged sufficiently, the resistance of the thin amnion to the pressure of the dorsal blastem fluid decreases. The thick ectoderm of the disc, as a result of the gradually increasing resistance of its basement membrane, then bends convexly towards the dorsal blastem fluid thereby forming an *expansion dome* (Expansionkuppe, Fig. 3-2, *see also* Chapter 4). This and similar findings indicate that the basement membrane, because of its qualities, also contributes substantially to differentiation. Even inconspicuous parts of the young organism appear to be important functional components of the whole embryo. This does not mean that such parts serve only one function and have a single importance. They can have extremely variable functions since the organism is an entirety in formal, physical and chemical dimensions.

As a result of the ectoderm arching into the dorsal blastem fluid, the cells in the expansion dome have an enlarged space towards the side of the fluid. The structure of these cells supports the principle that the superficial and basal sides of limiting tissue are connected by the cell limiting membranes in the shortest possible way, i.e. perpendicular. This alignment of the cell limiting membranes causes the cells to become wedge-shaped with the broad face directed towards the free surface of the expansion dome (divergent wedge epithelium). In accordance with this wedge shape of the cells, many nuclei migrate towards the free surface of the expansion dome. The cytoplasm in this area of the cells stains very lightly, indicating that it contains much water and has a relatively low viscosity. From regional comparisons, it is evident that nuclei in relatively liquid cytoplasm have the opportunity to move easily. Also their contained chromosomes tend to become mobile. The order of this phenomenon is another example of positional-dependent differentiation, i.e. of extragenetic information proceeding from the outside toward the inside. Evidently, in the region of divergent wedge epithelium, mitoses are most numerous near the free surface of the epithelium. When mitosis is complete, the "halved" daughter cells grow to normal size. They do so gradually, more and more assimilating from the basement membrane along their cell limiting membranes. In this way, surface growth of the wedge epithelium in the expansion dome is increased.

One could imagine the transition between chorionic mesoblast and covering mesoblast being a small point on the root of the body stalk (Fig. 3-2 above 2). Then, this zone should be interpreted as the chorionic pole on which the whole entocyst and its disc remain narrow (caudal end of the entocyst disc, Fig. 4-1). At the opposite end of the body stalk, the entocyst, as well as its disc, becomes broad. Here develops the obtuse, cranial end of the entocyst disc (Fig. 4-1). As this occurs, the growing expansion dome begins to biomechanically pull the adjacent endoderm. The cells in the inferior (caudal) part of the disc become compressed in a narrow area by the enlarging expansion dome. As a result, the entire disc bends into an S-shape during the third week (Fig. 3-2). The yolk sac gradually becomes an appendage of the disc and is structurally comparable to the anlage of an endocrine gland that gradually loses its duct (vitelline duct). The yolk sac possibly functions as a storage area that provides a constant supply of nourishment for the embryo when nourishment from the mother is temporarily reduced.

4

AXIAL PROCESS

As the entocyst disc undergoes an S-shaped bending, the embryo proper begins to be established. The bending initiates a folding that has very exact positional relationships. The cranial end of the disc is characterized by rapid growth. In contrast to this, growth of the caudal region is retarded. The limiting membranes of the ectodermal cells in the caudal region converge toward the free surface of the disc. The basement membrane underneath these cells does not expand. As a result, a depression or pit *(impansion pit,* Impansionssenke) forms in the ectoderm. This differentiation is in contrast to the expanded and domed ectoderm *(expansion dome)* in the cranial region of the disc (Fig. 4-1). In the region of the pit, ectoderm and endoderm are closely compressed with little space between them for the transport of nutritive substances along the basement membrane. The cells here are located in a region where evidently the conditions for growth are severely limited. Growth of the compressed ectoderm and endoderm in the floor of the pit is so reduced that a corrosion field is established *(see* Chapter 13). This region is the anlage of the cloacal membrane that later perforates.

The formation of positive and negative reliefs (expansion dome and impansion pit, respectively) in the entocyst disc is the

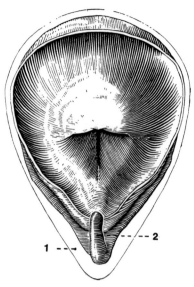

Figure 4-1. Entocyst disc, approximately 0.23 mm long, stage 6, approximately 13-14 days (Blechschmidt ovum, Carnegie no. 10318). Dorsal aspect showing the expansion dome (light) and impansion pit (central depressed area). *1*, area of the body stalk; *2*, allantois.

initial event that outlines the origin of the embryo. Usually, one is able to distinguish in the entocyst disc a broad cranial portion that has an obtuse shape, a narrow, trunk portion that is acutely shaped, and an important transition zone that represents the neck portion. The cranial portion is formed by the expansion dome. In the beginning of the third week, it makes up about half of the entocyst disc which was initially round and less than 0.5 mm in length. Caudally, the dome is so sharply continuous with the impansion pit that it appears half-moon-shaped (*see* upper part of the entocyst disc in Fig. 4-1). By comparing suitable stages, it becomes clear that cell multiplication and growth are less hindered toward the vertex of the "half-moon" than towards the lateral borders of the disc. The upper arrows in Figure 4-2 demonstrate the main, cranialward growth of the expansion dome on each side of the midline. This direction of growth is understandable, knowing where cell growth and multiplication are less hindered.

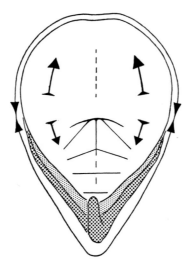

Figure 4-2. The dorsal aspect of the 0.23 mm entocyst disc showing growth movements. Divergent arrows represent main growth directions of the expansion dome. Convergent arrows indicate retarded growth of the marginal mesoblast. Anlage of the neural groove is shown by an interrupted midline in the dome area.

With these developmental movements, the disc loses its round shape as its head portion broadens progressively into a distinct, obtuse zone.   Lateral to the transition zone between expansion dome and impansion pit the border of the entocyst disc becomes straight (Fig. 4-2, convergent arrows).   This region will retract subsequently into a waist-like area of the embryo (Fig. 5-3).   During the third week, the (marginal) mesoblast bordering the entocyst disc becomes stretched as the "waist" develops. The meshwork of these mesodermal cells becomes longitudinally aligned in the same direction that it is stretched.   The stretch is caused by the mainly longitudinal growth of the disc.   The stretched meshwork outlines the path of the umbilical vein that arises at this time.

As the ectoderm is intensely growing in surface area in the region of the expansion dome, there is an enlargement of the distance between the rapidly growing ectoderm and the underlying endoderm.   Inner tissue similar in structure and origin to that of the mesoblast of the ovum arises between these two layers. As was previously seen, inner tissue arises when the surfaces of two adjacent, limiting tissues grow at different rates. On the cranial edge of the entocyst disc, the inner tissue forms a broad band between the epithelia of the two entoblast chambers (large stipple in Fig. 4-3 between *1* and *2*). This band forms the largest portion of the early middle blastoderm (mesoderm) and is present at the cranial umbilical border of the early entocyst disc. This mesoderm becomes loose as a result of the accumulation of extracellular substances. The process is similar to the loosening of the mesoblast of the ovum. Some of the intercellular substance apparently has been pressed out from the neighboring epithelia (ectoderm and endoderm). The two contacting epithelia seem to be pushed apart from each other by the liquid squeezing out.

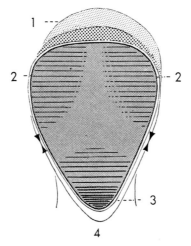

Figure 4-3. Drawing of the ventral aspect of the 0.23 mm entocyst disc. Endoderm is densely stippled. Large dots mark mesoderm. Convergent arrows represent the retarded growth of the marginal mesoblast. *1*, outer surface of amnion; *2*, cut edge of yolk sac; *3*, opening of the allantois; *4*, caudal umbilical border of the entocyst disc.

The mentioned term, inner tissue (Binnengewebe), is given to any cell aggregation that is deep to, and completely enclosed by limiting tissue (Grenzgewebe=epithelium). Limiting and limited (inner) tissues are distinguishable in the entocyst disc during the third week. The inner tissue becomes progressively loosened as the ectoderm of the broad region of the entocyst disc expands and overlaps the periphery of the ventral entoblast chamber or yolk sac (Fig. 4-3).

As a consequence of the arching of the expansion dome, the thick ectoderm is composed of wedge-shaped cells that vary in size from one area to another. Because of this, the surface growth rate of the ectoderm is not equal overall. Where divergence of the cell limiting membranes toward the free surface becomes extreme, the cytoplasm near the superficial cell limiting membranes is loosely arranged, has a high water content and exhibits an increased number of mitoses. Such an arrangement occurs particularly in the sharp transition between the expansion dome and the impansion pit.

Because the specific structure of the ectoderm varies from one location to another, growth of the ectoderm is unequal. This causes the area of the impansion pit to be overlapped by the caudal border of the expansion dome (Fig. 4-4, zone *1*). In other words, there is an abrupt transition in this region of the entocyst disc from a rapidly growing surface to a slowly growing surface. The so-called "rolled rim" area (Umbördelungsrand) is referred to in static terms as Hensen's node. In kinetic development it is an important differentiation zone forming the transition between rapid and slow growing areas of the entocyst disc. The formative function of this differentiation is the development of the *axial (notochordal) process*. It is the central part of the entocyst disc (Figs. 4-1 and 4-2).

Also, the axial process does not represent an isolated differentiation, which has originated from the interior, but it is a developmental dynamic component of the whole entocyst disc connected with all the differentiations at the periphery. When the axial process becomes distinct, the cranial and caudal ends, the dorsal and ventral sides and the left and right borders of the disc become established (*see* Chapters 2 and 3). What is later termed cranial and caudal, dorsal and ventral, and left and right results therefore from the developmental movements taking place within the ento-

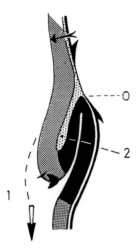

Figure 4-4. Transition between expansion dome and impansion pit showing the axial process of the 0.23 mm entocyst disc. Ectoderm is stippled. Axial process is solid black. Position of endoderm is represented by a heavy black line with convergent arrows showing retarded growth. Tailed arrow indicates the attraction of endoderm to ectoderm. Arrows near *1* show formation movements of ectoderm in the area of the rolling rim (Umbördelungsrand) of the expansion dome overlapping the impansion pit. *0*, tip of axial process; *2*, mesoderm.

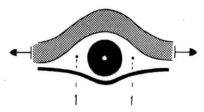

Figure 4-5. Axial process on transverse section. Ectoderm is stippled, endoderm is shown as heavy black line. Arrows show surface growth of ectoderm. *1*, mesoderm.

cyst disc. Generally, the above-mentioned developmental movements immediately result from the surface growth of the ectoderm. This growth is not a pure genetic process. Once again a developmental process is beginning externally and not in the nucleus (outside-inside differentiation) .

There is no doubt that the growth and consequently the metabolism of the axial process are less intense than they are for the expansion dome. Because of this phenomenon, the axial process gradually becomes of constructive importance for the origin and subsequent development of the embryo. Signs of growth resistance at the tip of the axial process have never been observed. If such a growth resistance occurred, it would be evident as cell aggregations that are aligned tangential to the end of the process, in a manner similar to waves leaving the bow of a boat as it moves through the water ("bow-waves"). Such waves would be expected if the axial process actively grew piston-like (as a Stemmkörper) into the space between the ectoderm and endoderm, separating the two layers as it moved. Actually, the cells at the tip of the process become loosely arranged to form mesoderm. This finding is a feature of longitudinal growth pull, which is a sign that the tip of the axial process itself is retarded in growth.

Topokinetic investigations do not support the notion that the axial process can be explained as a formation that is directed from within, without a required positional relationship given by its predevelopment.[5] The relatively slow growth of the axial process becomes evident during the early stages of development. Not only is its rate of lengthening slow but its diameter remains narrow at the same time. Initially, the process has the shape of a blind sac. Subsequently, it becomes tube-shaped. The lumen disappears during the third week and by the end of the week the notochord has been formed. At one time, the axial process had been interpreted as being a "head process." However, it is neither a "head process" nor the anlage of only the notochord for it also forms mesoderm.

That part of the expansion dome over the slow-growing axial process sinks below the surface, thereby forming the neural groove (Fig. 4-2, interrupted line in the middle of the dome). As the overlying ectoderm sinks, the endoderm comes into such close contact with the underside of the axial process that it gradually

---

[5]It is impossible to derive the human axial process from gastrulation that is observed in lower forms. In the zoological sense, a gastrula does not exist during human development. The term gastrulation has no meaning in human embryology.

fuses with the process (Figs. 4-4 and 4-5). As the neural groove arises, the wedge-epithelium that is laterally adjacent to it begins to protrude to form so-called "dorsal bulges" (Dorsalwulst). At first the bulges are only relative formations but eventually they become absolute and flank the neural groove. Their developmental kinetics are given in Chapter 5.

Because of the smallness of the axial process, the center of the early entocyst disc assumes kinetically remarkable importance. By its relatively slow growth, the axial process exerts formation functions by acting passively. By its restraining longitudinal growth, the process functions as a central regulator of surface growth of the entocyst disc. In this regard, one might say it is biodynamically a helper for the arising embryo. However, this does not mean that the axial process functions chemically in the sense of a so-called "inducer" or that it perhaps "makes" the development of other structures. The assumption that a central differentiation like the axial process has the potential to cause an effect from within itself is contrary to the observations. It is also contrary to the principle that *differentiations are directed primarily from the outside, inwards.* So that there are no misunderstandings, it is necessary to clarify at this particular time the following fact: *spontaneous, independent (selbsttätig) inducers do not exist in the chemical sense.*

5

THE EARLY EMBRYO

A PRINCIPLE MENTIONED EARLIER needs to be restated at this time, namely, *at any particular moment during development, an organism functions according to the features its organs have attained at that time.* Even during and because of its development, each organ, that is, each body part that can be isolated by dissection, contributes to the formation of the whole organism. This means that each organ of the body has forming or formative functions from its very beginning. Consequently, from its very beginning each organ performs work. In this sense, static and functionless organs cannot be demonstrated. Therefore, this is one good reason to consider all differentiations in their early stages of development as being functionally important, even though they are hardly visible and may have previously received little or no attention.

From the above statements one would expect early human embryos to have formative functions also. The formative functions of embryos can be determined from their developmental movements. In the preceeding chapter the axial process was shown to have considerable biodynamic importance. Actually, its development causes the neural groove to form. According to its position and shape, the growth of the axial process is retarded. Since the overlying ectoderm is closely attached to the process, the process exerts a growth resistance against this ectoderm causing its growth to also become retarded (Fig. 5-1). In this manner the axial process is important in the construction of the early embryo. Formation of the neural groove gives rise to dorsal bulges that appear on each side of the groove and become longitudinal folds. Establishment of the neural groove causes the cell limiting membranes of the wedge epithelium (Keilepithel) covering the dorsal bulges to become increasingly divergent. This divergence is directed toward the amniotic cavity (Fig. 5-2, divergent lines).

From Blechschmidt's investigations it has been concluded that longitudinal growth of the dorsal bulges is caused by the divergence of the epithelial cells of the dorsal bulges. It happens in the following manner. The radius of each bulge is less in transverse section than it is in longitudinal section. In other words, each bulge curves more in the transverse plane than in the longitudinal plane (Fig. 5-3). On transverse section, the cell limiting membranes diverge considerably toward the surface. On the other hand, in the longitudinal plane (longer bulge radius) the limiting membranes of the epithelial cells are aligned nearly parallel to one another. From this, one sees that the three-dimensional shape of the mentioned epithelial cells is prism-like (Fig. 5-4). As mentioned above, opportunity for mitosis is great near the free surface. The new cells produced by mitosis grow towards their nutrients thereby penetrating into the depth because the nutrients of the cells are located at the base of the ectoderm. The movement is easier in the intercellular interstices along the transverse plane of the dorsal bulges than along their longitudinal planes. By these developmental movements the new cells contribute crucially to the lengthening of the embryo.

By comparing developmental movements in different regions, one finds a similar arrangement in other longitudinally growing tissues. Examples of such tissues are early embryonic tubules and epithelial edges such as the marginal ridge of limb buds. The epithelial cells on all of these tissues are prism-shaped (wedge epithelium) and, consequently, the tissue grows mainly in a longitudinal direction. Thus, the axial process causes the arising of the neural groove and, as a consequence of its origin, the forma-

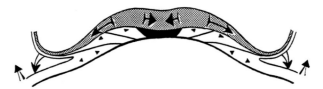

Figure 5-1. Illustration of an entocyst (trilaminar) disc on transverse section (Heuser embryo, 1.25 mm, stage 8, 18 days, Carnegie no. 5960). Medially, surface growth of the ectoderm over the axial process (solid black area) is hindered (convergent arrows). The lateral outlined arrows indicate the unrolling of the lateral body wall. The divergent arrows with base lines show surface growth of the ectoderm. Arrowheads represent the fluid pressure of the intercellular substance.

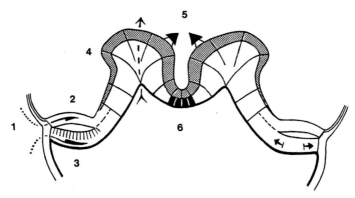

Figure 5-2. Illustration of the Ludwig embryo on transverse section (1.8 mm, stage 9, 21 days, Carnegie no. 5982) showing the principal alignments of the cell limiting membranes. Upper arrows show the movement establishing the neural tube. The arrow with a broken line indicates permeation. Lateral half-headed arrows indicate the parathelial supply of nutrients from the chorionic cavity. Katabolites are released into the coelomic cavity. *1,* lateral umbilical border; *2,* ectoderm of the early embryonic "thoracic wall" corresponding to the lateral arching shown in Figure 5-3 at level *1; 3,* endoderm of the early embryonic "thoracic wall;" *4,* dorsal bulge; *5,* neural groove; *6,* axial process.

tion of the dorsal bulges. In this way the axial process gives rise indirectly to the longitudinal growth of the early anlage of the embryo.

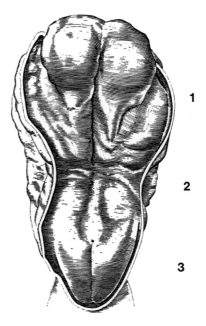

Figure 5-3. Dorsal aspect of the Ludwig embryo showing its cranial *1*, cervical *2* and trunk *3* subdivisions.

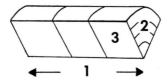

Figure 5-4. Diagram showing the prism-shape of wedge epithelium cells (of the dorsal bulge). *1*, main growth direction of the dorsal bulge (lengthening growth); *2*, transverse plane; *3*, longitudinal plane.

As is known, the medial slope of the dorsal bulges greatly thickens and forms the epithelial anlage of the nervous system while the lateral slope becomes relatively thin and forms the anlage of the body wall of the cranial, cervical and trunk regions (Figs. 5-2 and 5-3, levels *1, 2, 3*). The first result of the longitudinal growth of the bulges is the stretching of the adjacent mesoblast in the early umbilical region. As the mesoblast accommodates the expanding ectoderm, the "neck" of the early embryo is formed. The initiation of these developmental movements is shown with convergent arrows in Figure 4-2. These movements bring about the sandal shape of the approximately 1.8 mm embryo (Fig. 5-3).

In Chapter 3 it was shown that the ectodermal surface of the entocyst disc expands at a more rapid rate than the endodermal surface. This indicates that the ectoderm, which is the strongest part of the early embryo, is the structure primarily responsible for its formation. The question then arises as to how the ectoderm receives its necessary nutrients. Without the assimilation of nutritive substances, growth of the ectoderm would be impossible. It was previously seen that ectodermal cells are polarized according to the thickness of the ectoderm which, in turn, depends on the position of the ectoderm during development. As a result of polarization, ectodermal cells probably assimilate nutrients from the region of the basement membrane and release watery katabolites (dissimilate) on their free surface.

Studies on serial sections clearly show that the endoderm does not keep pace with the intense surface growth of the ectoderm. In comparison with ectoderm, growth of the endoderm is retarded. Because of this, the distance between ectoderm and endoderm increases. As the distance increases, mesoderm arises as a mesh-like aggregation of cells in the space between the two limiting (epithelial) tissues that grow at different rates (Fig. 5-1). Similar developmental kinetics were seen for the origin of the mesoblast.

As development proceeds, the amniotic cavity enlarges in relation to the total volume of the conceptus, whereas the yolk-sac becomes smaller. Consideration of these facts suggests that the mesoderm is kinetically important for the differentiation of the entocyst disc. As the axial process and dorsal bulges form, the mesodermal cells adapt to the surface growth of the ectoderm by aligning perpendicularly between the ectoderm and the endoderm. The larger part of the cell containing the nucleus does not lie immediately adjacent to the ectoderm or endoderm. Only the tips of thin processes of the mesodermal cells attach to the endoderm and ectoderm. Fluid intercellular substance collects in the wide spaces between the cell processes. This conforms to the usual finding that inner tissues congest katabolites in the cell interstices since limiting tissues release them by the shortest way, i.e. perpendicular to their surface. The limiting membranes of the cell processes enclosing the fluid intercellular substance form a system of trajectories (Fig. 5-2). Fluid in the interior of the mesoderm are sites of biomechanical pressure. Likewise, the cell limiting membranes are sites of biomechanical tensile stress. The distribution of the stress certainly implicates chemical metabolic processes. Already in the third week, the cell interstices form the spaces for vascularization, particularly for the arising capillary anlagen of the aortae (Fig. 6-1). The vascularization shows once again the regularity of developmental movements which evidently indicate spatially directed, metabolic movements.

Metabolic movements have been repeatedly mentioned as having an orderly arrangement in space. Now it should be added that during early development their spatial order is based on the given structures. Such structures have a trajectorial arrangement and exhibit main directions of the growth tension on membranes. They also exhibit the principal alignment of intercellular gaps where molecular nutrients and katabolites move according to metabolic gradients. A diffuse distribution of nutrients does not occur in the early embryo. It would be reasonable for the pathways through which nutrients for the ovum and early embryo are distributed to be arranged according to the principal directions of the trajectorial system. Such an arrangement is compatible with other findings.

During the second week the ectoderm and endoderm probably receive nutrients by way of their basement membrane. The nutrients appear to come mostly from the equator region of the ovum. At the beginning of the third week, when the chorionic cavity is formed but the body-stalk vessels have not yet formed, nourishment probably comes from the entire chorion into the interior of the entocyst. The entocyst is the central metabolic field of the young ovum. Here nutrients are absorbed from the chorionic cavity by the yolk sac, and katabolites are returned from the amniotic cavity through the amnion into the chorionic cavity towards the chorion. By the third week, when sufficient mesoderm has been formed in the entocyst disc, the distribution of the submicroscopic nutrients probably occurs by means of the mesoderm parallel to the limiting tissues. This subject will be discussed further in Chapter 6.

During the third week the mesenchyma of the body stalk is already composed of communicating cell interstices. The arrangement of the mesenchyma is in accordance with a metabolic field that has an orderly arrangement in space. All of the cellular interstices are aligned longitudinally in the direction of the body stalk. The channel for the umbilical vein passes in the mesenchyma on the dorsal side of the body stalk. At the same time, the paired aortae leave the anlage of the embryo and pass to the interstices for the umbilical arteries on the ventral side of the stalk. The anlagen of the umbilical arteries being part of the body stalk cause it to arch convexly into the chorionic cavity. This demonstrates that arteries with their higher pressure lengthen at a faster rate than do the weaker, low-pressure veins. This observation is in accordance with a rule for the development of blood vessels. It is believed that the bending of the body stalk is caused by the restraining function of the unpaired umbilical vein against the umbilical arteries in the stalk. If this were not true, then one would expect the arteries to be straight because of their higher blood pressure.

Since the intercellular substance in the early ectoderm is not congested, no vessels would be expected to develop in it. Early ectoderm probably has no currents within it that move in opposite directions. Assimilation and dissimilation in opposite directions initiate the formation of arteries and veins. The ectodermal layer may be a "one-way," polarized metabolic field that releases katabolites on its free surface and assimilates substances on the side covered by mesoderm.

By examining the position, shape and structure of the mesoderm with this in view and by comparing Figs. 5-1 and 5-2, the changes one observes in the early embryo can be explained. Only the ectodermal (dorsal) limiting tissue is thick. A study of the developmental movement reveals that the expanding ectodermal surface encounters more resistance medially in the region of the neural groove (near the axial process) than it does laterally. It may be concluded that because of the growth resistance encountered medially, the ectoderm thickens more medially than laterally.

This introduces another principle of differentiation, namely, *when epithelium (limiting tissue) is hindered in its ability to expand (surface growth), it becomes thicker.* The thickened ectoderm rolls inward medially, but laterally it rolls outward. The biodynamic explanation of this is that the lateral, outward rolling of the ectoderm is caused by retarded growth of the adjacent mesoblast that surrounds the umbilical region while the amnion continues to enlarge (Figs. 5-1 and 5-2).

As the tissues in the region of the cranial umbilical edge increase in thickness, the mesoderm following the surface growth of the limiting tissues becomes loose and gives rise to the appearance of the intraembryonic coelomic cavity. This process is similar to the formation of the chorionic (mesoblast) cavity. The development of this portion of the coelomic cavity is immediately important for the appearance of the heart anlage.

Spherical-shaped vacuolations gradually expand in the mesoderm and form the left and right pleuropericardial cavities. They approach each other medially. The mesenchyma between the right and left cavities is arranged as a roughly X-shaped band. This band is the anlage of the heart in embryos approximately 2 mm in length (Figs. 5-5 to 5-7). The characteristic origin of the heart anlage is determined by its position. This is another example of the concept that differentiation movements begin external to any given region, and effect changes from there inwards, not vice versa. When the two expanding anlagen of the coelom (early pleuropericardial cavity) join each other ventrally, the X-shaped heart anlage enlarges as the neural tube enlarges. Enlargement of the heart anlage is closely related to expansion of the brain portion of the neural tube. The heart anlage then appears as a fold-like protrusion on the dorsal wall of the coelomic (pleuropericardial) cavity of the early embryo and is almost vertical in its alignment (Fig. 5-7).

This positional development of the heart determines the shape

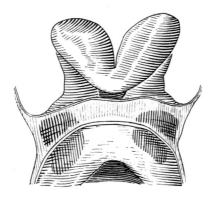

Figure 5-5. Drawing of the ventral aspect of the cranial region of an early embryo (Davis embryo, 4 somites, stage 10, 22 days, Carnegie no. 3709). Lateral parts of the anlage of the early pleuropericardial cavity are cross-hatched.

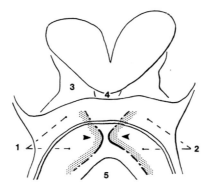

Figure 5-6. Diagram corresponding to Fig. 5-5. Broken lines represent the principal alignment of the mesenchyma between the paired pleuropericardial cavity of the early embryo that has an X-shaped heart anlage. *1* and *2,* sites of the bilateral early embryonic pleuropericardial cavities in the mesoderm of the cranial umbilical border. *3,* right first pharyngeal arch; *4,* oropharyngeal membrane; *5,* cranial (upper) intestinal portal. Arrowheads represent the fluid pressure in the cavities.

of the heart. Initially, the heart is almost bilaterally symmetrical. At the end of the third week, the intercellular substance of the heart mesenchyma seems to be gradually influenced by the metabolic gradient that comes from the terminal part of the umbilical

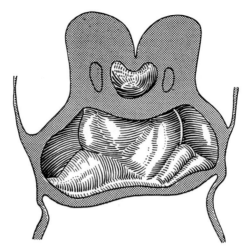

Figure 5-7. Drawing of the same embryo shown in Figure 5-5 with the ventral wall of the early thorax anlage removed. The X-shaped heart anlage is thereby exposed lying against the dorsal wall.

veins located at the caudal border of the heart anlage. This metabolic gradient is directed toward the very cellular epithelium of the brain anlage where the nutritive substances are assimilated. A capillary channel subsequently develops in the heart anlage and protrudes ventrally in the direction of least resistance. Fluid will flow into the capillary channel at the caudal side of the anlage and will flow out the cranial side. In accordance with its X-shape the heart anlage has a paired afferent pathway caudally and a paired efferent pathway cranially. The capillary channels communicate with each other by an unpaired connection. The connecting area is the most mobile part of the heart anlage. It bends more and more asymmetrically[6] and fills the entire pleuropericardial cavity. The heart, which at this time is still a capillary, is the primary organ of the pleuropericardial cavity of the early embryo.

[6]Bilateral symmetry in the mathematical sense never exists in human development. One can show that even during the early stages of development the dorsal and ventral chambers of the entocyst never lie directly over one another in the region cranial to the umbilical edge of the early embryo anlage. The dorsal chamber usually lies more toward the left (Fig. 4-3). This asymmetry is perpetuated throughout development.

At this particular time during development there is probably a large osmotic pressure difference between the fluid in the capillary heart anlage (blood) and the fluid in the early pleuropericardial cavity (serous fluid). The pressure difference causes a dilation of the wall of the still weak heart anlage thereby giving rise to dilation of the heart tube, the greatest part of which is bending initially in the ventral direction. The afferent and efferent pathways are progressively distinguishable as being bent in a dorsal direction. These bendings all together form a loop that is almost Ω-shaped in the lateral view. The loop is S-shaped on its ventral aspect. The cardiac musculature which originates in dilation fields during expansion of the early heart wall will be discussed in Chapter 18.

During further differentiation, the paired afferent vessels at the caudal end of the heart anlage (inflow path) become more transverse in their alignment in accordance with the transverse positioning of the cranial edge of the umbilical region. The paired efferent vessels at the cranial end of the heart anlage (outflow path) become longitudinally straight and lengthen as the brain anlage lengthens. When they straighten in the longitudinal direction, they come to lie immediately lateral to the mouth anlage in the sort of "cheeks" of the early embryo (Fig. 5-7). These developmental movements are prerequisites for the direction of the blood stream. When the cardiac musculature becomes contractile (contractibility is a reaction to initial dilation), the blood is thereby propelled toward the aortic anlagen because they are aligned in the direction of least resistance.

Attention will now be turned to neural groove closure. What developmental movements bring this about? Closure begins in the narrowest part of the entocyst disc in its so-called "cervical" portion (Fig. 5-3, level 2). Narrowing of the disc causes the borders of the neural groove to approach each other in a particular way. Closure involves the rolling-in of the neural groove borders. The following principle explains how this would occur. After the neural groove and the dorsal bulges appear, the cell limiting membranes of the latter diverge toward the free surface. This arrangement is especially evident in the transverse plane where the neural epithelium becomes continuous with the body wall epithelium (Fig. 5-2). The cell limiting membrane at the free surface (outer black line in Fig. 5-2) expands as the epithelium becomes wedge-shaped and diverges. From this it is apparent that the wedge shape of the cells is caused by a broadening of the free surface side of the cells so that the now narrow end forms an apex or tip. The cytoplasm just beneath the superficial cell limiting membrane is not very dense. This suggests that the water produced by metabolism is retained and increased by osmosis in this part of the cells causing the cytoplasm to be loosely arranged. The nuclei migrate from the relatively narrow (deep) side of the cells into the loose cytoplasm located in the more superficial part of the cells. Here, the nuclei have a greater outer and inner mobility resulting in a higher mitotic rate. The nucleus may move easily in the watery part of the cell, and its inner substances (chromosomes) may change their position and shape in the nucleus when loosely arranged. When mitosis is over, the daughter cells displace towards the basement membrane and increase due to nutrients from the stroma. As this growth occurs, the surface of the neural epithelium in contact with the underlying stroma becomes more enlarged than the free surface. In this way, the neural groove closes (Fig. 5-2) establishing the neural tube. However, this process is only understandable when, at the same time, the floor of the neural tube exerts a growth resistance. Indeed, in the floor of the neural groove, very few mitoses can be found. The basement membrane is relatively strong. Here fluid appears to be pressed out of the cytoplasm and the nuclei are relatively immobile. The growth rate is very slow in this region.

Closure of the neural groove at the cranial end of the embryo requires a somewhat different process since the head region bends during development causing the neuropore to widen (Fig. 5-8). This area resembles the gaping of a cut in the skin over the joint of a flexed finger. Because of this phenomenon, the cranial neuropore closes slowly. The wedge epithelium in the lateral edge of the neuropore becomes extremely divergent toward the free surface. Water again accumulates in the cytoplasm at the wide, free surface end of the wedge-shaped cells. The cell nuclei migrate towards the free surface. The low viscosity of the cytoplasm in this region possibly causes an intensive outer and inner mobility of the nucleus. The inner mobility (movements of chromosomes) allows inner structures to change. Such a phenomenon could explain the increase in mitoses that occurs near fluid (ventricular). After mitosis the new cells migrate toward the deep side of the neural epithelium which is contacting the stroma (Fig. 5-10A, *1*). The migrating and growing cells would cause the deep surface of the neural epithelium to expand (origin of the optic vesicle). As this occurred, the edge of the neuropore would roll in, leading gradually to closure of the neuropore (Figs. 5-9 and 5-10).

In normally bent embryos, approximately 2.5 mm in length, the cranial part of the neural groove is still open. The optic sulcus gradually forms in this open segment as a deep recess in the

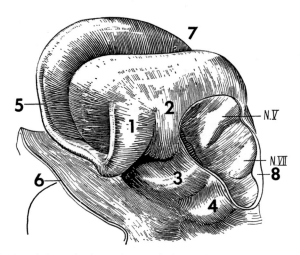

Figure 5-8. Craniolateral view of the Blechschmidt embryo (3.1 mm, 13 somites, stage 11, 24 days, Carnegie no. 10304). *1*, Serial section reconstruction; *1*, embryonic eye anlage; *2*, maxillary bulge (upper jaw of the embryo); *3*, mandibular bulge (lower jaw of the embryo); *4*, hyoid bulge (hypolingual arch); *5*, optic sulcus at entrance to optic vesicle anlage; *6*, cut edge of amnion; *7*, cranial neuropore; *8*, otic placode. Part of lateral ectoderm is cut away showing the position of the trigeminal (N. V) and facioacoustic (N. VII) nerve anlagen. Real facial processes have never been observed. They do not exist (Hochstetter, 1897).

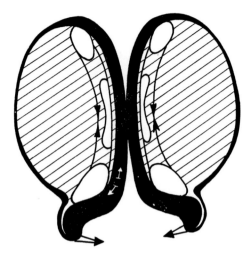

Figure 5-9. Illustration of a horizontal section through the border of the cranial neuropore of the same 3.1 mm embryo shown in Figure 5-8. Biokinetics of the tissue is shown with arrows. Divergent arrows represent rapid expansion growth of the neural epithelium. Convergent arrows represent retarded growth of the adjacent blood vessels. Outlined arrows show initial closing of the cranial neuropore in the eye region.

area where the third ventricle later develops (Fig. 5-8). The sulcus is the opening of the optic ventricle of the early embryo (1973, pp. 10 and 15). From the biokinetic view, the optic sulcus is caused by the initial broadening of the early embryonic brain. As soon as the cranial neuropore closes, a corrosion field *(see* Chapter 13) is established in the area of closure. The epithelial cells in this field perish. As a result, the neural epithelium separates from the adjacent ectoderm. As the junction line disappears, the optic vesicles appear as appendages of the diencephalic part of the prosencephalon. They are the first blind, lateral extensions of the prosencephalon and are similar to the cerebral hemispheres (vesicles) that develop later.

From the biodynamic viewpoint, the edge of the cranial neuropore is an important structure in the initiation of the ear as well as the eye. As the neuropore widens during the initial bending of the embryonic head, the ectoderm at the caudal border of the

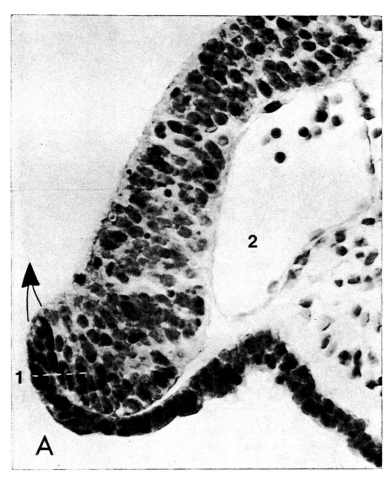

Figure 5-10 A and B. (*A*) A horizontal section through the cranial region of the same 3.1 mm embryo shown in Figure 5-8. 800×. *1,* transition of ectoderm into neural epithelium; *2,* vein. *(B)* Diagram of the section showing developmental movements in the transition zone between ectoderm and neural epithelium. Large outlined arrow shows direction of movement for neuropore closure at the border of the optic sulcus. Small outlined arrow indicates direction of cell migration. Divergent arrows represent intense growth of neural epithelium. The relatively slow growth of the superficial ventricular surface of the neural epithelium is shown by convergent arrows. Lowest arrow shows surface growth of ectoderm. Horizontal arrow with interrupted stem indicates the restraining function of the vein (unlabelled in Fig. 5-9).

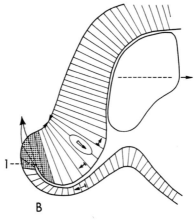

Figure 5-10B.

neuropore becomes compressed and consequently thickens (Fig. 5-8, *8*) (1961, p. 309). It is in this manner that the otic placode forms. The ear and the eye appear in the region of the cranial neuropore as biodynamic modifications of the differentiating epithelium. In other words, they are parts of the external modifications of the growing embryo.

The general relationships in these two areas cannot be explained by the commonly used term "induction." "Induction" refers only to possible chemical influences on development. Developmental kinetics explains the movements that occur much better than do "chemicals." However, this is not to deny that it is possible to describe conclusively an organism with other points of view.

6

SOMITES

Potentialities are potentialities only under certain circumstances. When the capabilities of developmental potentialities of a particular region of the embryo are discussed, it is meant that the region always has these potentialities under certain circumstances. Therefore it is important to discuss the circumstances of cell aggregations. It would be meaningless to discuss their potentialities divorced from their positional relationships. Consequently, before normal differentiation processes can be correlated, one must know the exact position of the metabolic fields in which the differentiation takes place. Experimental analyses alone, without consideration of the particular circumstances brought about by specific positional relationships, cannot possibly give an adequate view of *normal* differentiation processes.

Studies on the position of developmental movements (topokinesis) have lead to the following principle: *The potentialities of every organ during development are in accordance with the features the organ shows as the result of its positional relationships.* This means that close attention should be given to the fact that the potentialities of an area change with each step of development. The developmental origin of somites is a prime example of this principle. A specific cytoplasm already present in the ovum is also the prerequisite for establishing somites. For its differentiating function this cytoplasm requires extragenetic information from the cell limiting membrane and genetic information from the nucleus for each stage of predevelopment.

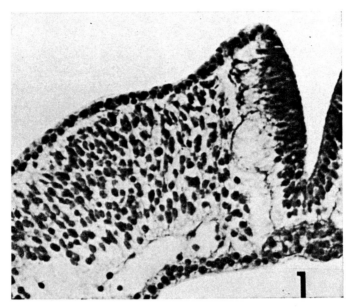

Figure 6-1. Transverse section of the Blechschmidt embryo (3.1 mm, 13 somites, stage 11, approximately 24 days). 390×. Section is through unsegmented mesoderm at the level of the caudal neuropore. The site of the aorta is visible along the endoderm which forms gut roof *(1)*.

What are somites from the kinetic viewpoint? Neither comparative anatomical observations nor experimental investigations can show the origin of the processes that bring about somite formation and the resulting segmentation (metamerism). However, the morphological findings can be explained biokinetically. Just prior to somite formation, unsegmented inner tissue (mesoderm) is located dorsolateral to the caudal neuropore between neural epithelium and the extraembryonic coelom (Fig. 6-1). This unsegmented inner tissue transforms into somites (Fig. 6-2). Somites first appear on about the twenty-third day as thick-walled vesicles. The dorsal part of the vesicle wall lies near the ectoderm. It is very cellular and will later give rise to the dermatome. The ventral part of the wall lies near the endoderm and dorsal aorta anlage. This zone contains abundant intercellular substances and subsequently gives rise to the sclerotome (Fig. 6-2).

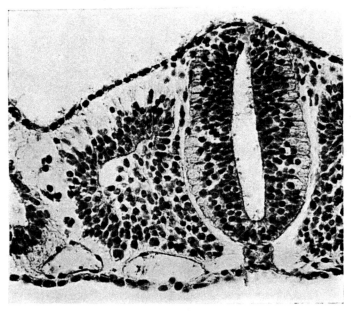

Figure 6-2. Transverse section of the same embryo shown in Figure 6-1. Section is through the region of a somite. 270×.

Each vesicle is surrounded by a capsule. Segmentation septa represent early portions of the capsule and are best observed in sagittal sections. The ventral portion or base of each septum is relatively thick and is composed of many densely packed cells. The somites located between the segmentation septa are correspondingly small ventrally and broad dorsally. The cells of each somite are dense dorsally and loose ventrally and are aligned perpendicular to the capsule. Accordingly, they are arranged in a radial manner around the cavity of the somite which is temporarily free of cells (Figs. 6-2 and 6-4). This radial arrangement allows the cell limiting membranes to unite the inner and outer surfaces of the somite wall in the shortest way possible. Comparison of very young embryos reveals a remarkable uniformity in the location of cytoplasm and nuclei in the walls of early hollow organs. At the beginning of the third week, nuclei are always crowded near the cavity whereas thin processes of the cell bodies are located more peripheral to the cavity, near the basement membrane of the limiting tissues.

From the foregoing, it may be seen that each somite has a particular position, shape and structure. At each stage, development of a somite is part of the development of the whole embryo. Therefore, the movements that are described for the position, shape and structure of somites during development must be consistent with the movements occurring in the whole embryo. What are these movements?

Somites are known to arise from unsegmented mesenchyma that has a characteristic structure. When the intercellular fluid increases in volume, the mesenchymal cells align perpendicular to the ectoderm and endoderm (Fig. 6-1). The cells assume this position because the perpendicular alignment is the position of least resistance when the intercellular fluid increases. The biodynamics of this phenomenon was interpreted previously when the early germ layers were examined (*see* Chapter 5). This biodynamic interpretation will now be reexamined. The intercellular fluid is the site of biomechanical pressure forces. On the other hand, the cell limiting membranes are the site of biomechanical tensile stresses. Here also, cell alignment is associated with a strongly ordered arrangement of the intercellular fluid. Intercellular fluid is very abundant ventrally, near the endoderm, but sparse dorsally, near the ectoderm.

The biodynamic interpretation of this phenomenon is shown in the diagram in Figure 6-3. As a result of the developing shape of the embryo, the ectodermal surface expands more than the endodermal surface, obviously because the surface of the ectoderm grows more intensely. Because of this, there is more space for the large mesenchymal cell bodies and nuclei near the ectoderm than near the endoderm. Many narrow, tapered cell processes are located near the endoderm. Intercellular fluid collects between these tapered portions of the cells giving the area a congested appearance (Fig. 6-1). It seems reasonable to conclude from this arrangement that the mesenchymal cells do not have as strong a contact with the endoderm as they do with the ectoderm. In general, the contact area between the mesenchymal cell bodies and the ectoderm is broader and closer than the contact areas are between the tapered processes of the mesenchymal cells and the endoderm. The broad connections between the ectoderm and adjacent mesenchyma are not connections of a mechanical kind. It would be more natural for them to be living metabolic connections. Support for this is the fact that cell limiting membranes are very thin, as permeable membranes are known to be. With sufficient magnification, fluid is visible between the limiting tissues and the inner tissue which is counter to the suggestion that these cells "stick together."

Findings support the concept that particles of the metabolic cycle move along the basement membrane particularly of the endoderm. Support of this concept is the fact that the first blood vessels arise in the vicinity of the endoderm and are not found in any other location (Figs. 6-1 and 6-2). From what has been said, the adjacent germ layers could be viewed as layers that are closely connected by their metabolic activity. There is no reason for the assumption that intercellular fluid stagnates; on the contrary, it is continually flowing. Probably the metabolic movements in the mesenchyma occur not in two but in three dimensions. Therefore we have shown the movements to be aligned parallel and perpendicular to membranes (arrows in Fig. 6-3).

Figure 6-4 is a diagram of the position, shape and structure of somites as they arise from unsegmented paraxial mesenchyma. The purpose of this diagram is to provide an overall view of the movements that accompany the developmental origin of somites. The diagram was taken from serial sections. The main direction of the cells in the unsegmented mesenchyma is perpendicular to the ectoderm and endoderm (Fig. 6-1). This arrangement is seen near the caudal end of the embryo and is indicated in Figure 6-4 (lower part) by several straight lines. Such unsegmented mesenchyma is regularly found in the area of establishing seg-

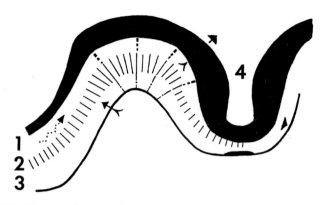

Figure 6-3. Diagram showing the general arrangement of the cells in Figure 5-2. *1*, lightly staining zone; *2*, darkly staining zone with nuclei; *3*, lightly staining zone that has abundant intercellular material; *4*, neural groove. Arrows indicate metabolic movements which occur along epithelia (parathelial) and perpendicular through epithelia (diathelial).

mentation. The Ludwig embryo shows such a zone bilaterally in the waist-shaped body region (Fig. 5-3) where the embryo is "lordotic." Here the first pair of segmentation furrows appear just after the mesenchymal anlagen of the aortae have established bilaterally in the mesenchyma. In this zone the mesenchyma is deprived of nutrients for the growing neural epithelium.

Branches of the dorsal aorta grow following the metabolic gradient towards the neural epithelium at close craniocaudal intervals. This is an important initiation of segmentation. In accordance with the general rule of blood vessel development, the aortic branches do not elongate rapidly enough to keep pace with the surrounding tissue. The branches thereby remain relatively short. This causes the overlying ectoderm to be more and more retracted into a segmentation furrow. It should be pointed out at this time that generally blood vessels do not grow on their own accord but are stimulated to grow where there exists a need for nutrients. Blood vessels grow according to their position in relation to this need. From observations, the authors have been led to believe that the origin of the dorsal metameric branches of the aortae is caused by a metabolic gradient between the aorta and the neural tube in the area of the caudal neuropore where the tube is growing appositionally. In this region, there is an intense branching or sprouting of the aortae in the caudal direction. These branches not only supply the neural tube but also the ectoderm and the neighboring tissue. Intersegmental veins complete the explained development.

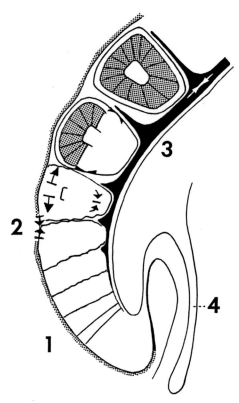

Figure 6-4. Diagram of a paramedian section through a reconstruction of the same embryo in Figure 6-1 showing some of the biokinetic features of somite development. Divergent arrows with base lines represent growth near the ectoderm. Convergent simple arrows indicate cells compressed between the metameric aortic branches. Convergent arrows with base lines show retarded growth. Convergent arrows indicate the restraining function of the somite capsule and aorta. *1,* still unsegmented dorsal region deficient in blood vessels; *2,* segmentation furrow; *3,* gut region with neighboring aorta (black); *4,* allantois.

As the neural groove begins to close the edge of the neural groove in the transition area between neural and body wall ectoderm becomes progressively sharper. The ectodermal cells diverge in a fan-like manner medialwards, their nuclei are displaced towards the surface where they undergo mitosis. The subsequently enlarging daughter cells form the somite bulge. As the ectodermal cells of the somite bulge diverge towards the free surface, the cells in the area of the segmentation furrow converge towards the free surface. However, these latter cells diverge with their broad side towards the notochord and the aorta anlagen. Thus, the ectoderm grows unequally and is followed by the mesenchyma. It grows slowly together with the blood vessels under the segmentation furrows forming the segmentation septa, but under the bulges it grows more rapidly. When the caudal (lower) neuropore migrates caudalwards the first pair of somites succeed caudally the first paired segmentation septum. The first pair of somites is bordered by the second pair of segmentation septa. This differentiation proceeds caudalwards as the embryo in the fourth week becomes more and more lengthened caudally. When compared with the bending folds of the embryo (the pharyngeal arches) the arising segments become established as being straightening folds. The bent lower part of the body is straightened by the blood pressure of the aorta, which is growing caudalwards.

As the bending of the embryo increases and the neural groove closes, the somites broaden more dorsally than they do ventrally (Figs. 6-2 and 6-4). Conversely, the segmentation septa between the somites become narrow dorsally, and broader ventrally. As a result, the somites and septa appear as alternating wedges joined to each other.

The cavity of the somite is a metabolic field that is comparable to the neurocoele and coelomic cavity of the young embryo. Katabolites, especially water, are located in the cavities and are drained by the cell interstices and veins. The zone where nutrients are assimilated is peripheral to the cavities. It is interesting that mitoses in somites are not synchronous with mitoses in adjacent tissue. Since mitoses are asynchronous it can be concluded that growth of the tissues occurs at different rates. At any given moment, small portions of the somite expand more rapidly than do adjacent tissues (ectoderm and segmentation septa) and thereby slide against them. The somitic capsule probably arises as a result of these sliding movements. Histological studies show that processes of the somitic cells bend into the capsule and align tangential to the surface of the somite. Such an alignment should be expected when sliding movements occur. As soon as the capsule has enlarged and strengthened sufficiently, it acts as a restraining apparatus (Fig. 6-4, convergent arrows at periphery of somites). In general, this is a typical function of capsules. Somitic cells at the periphery flatten and align tangential to the surface of the somite. Because of this, it is concluded that the expanding somite exerts growth pressure thereby causing a restraining function of the capsule which gives rise to a round configuration of the somites. Thereby they give space to the dorsal branches of the aortae for enlarging along the neural tube (Fig. 6-5).

Cells in the dorsal part of the somite near the ectoderm increase in number causing the somite to thicken. This portion is the dermatome. Cells in the deep ventral part of the somite have less room for expanding and are less numerous. This part of the somite narrows in the region between the neural tube and the mesonephros and becomes the sclerotome (Fig. 6-6). A segmentation septum is located just cranial and caudal to the micrographic section in Figure 6-6. The basal (ventral) part of the septum contains many nuclei and consequently stains dark in histological sections. It soon becomes distinct as the anlage of an intervertebral disc. The sclerotome and segmentation septum can not be clearly distinguished from each other. The cells comprising both structures blend ventrally and medially with the tissue around the neural tube and notochord. In Chapter 9 the way the neural tube also becomes metamerically arranged will be explained.

The bodies of the vertebral column always develop from the light-staining sclerotomes that are located *medial to* the dorsal branches of the aorta. At the beginning of the second month the cells in these regions appear vesicular and represent the anlagen of the vertebral bodies, the first cartilaginous anlagen to form.

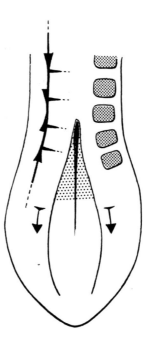

Figure 6-5. Diagram of the dorsal aspect of the lower trunk end of the same embryo shown in Figure 6-1. The segmentation zone shows segmentation folds (densely stippled) and segmentation furrows in an alternating arrangement. The metameric branches of the paired aorta are located beneath the ectoderm of the furrows. They are structures representing tension stresses. Convergent arrows show the restraining function of aorta and metameric branches. Arrows with base lines indicate the growth expansion of the ectoderm along the neural tube. Caudal neuropore is coarsely stippled.

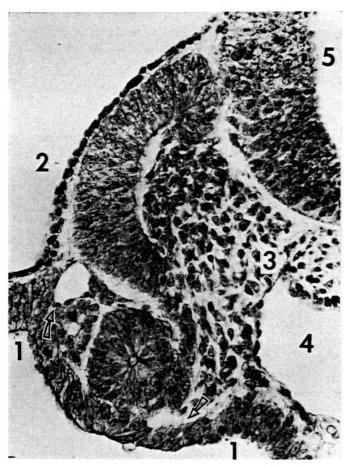

Figure 6-6. Transverse section of a 3.4 mm embryo (Blechschmidt), 27 somites, stage 12, approximately 27 days, (Carnegie no. 10306). 370×. Section is through the caudal part of the embryo. Tissue between *1* and *1* is the region of the retrositus. Laterally, between the arrows, is the mesonephric (Wolffian) duct, medially, the anlage of a mesonephric tubule; *2*, dermatome; *3*, sclerotome; *4*, the unpaired dorsal aorta; *5*, neurocoel. Arrows show the rotary movement of tissue around a longitudinal axis in the region of the retrositus (*see* text).

Intervertebral discs develop in the area of the basal part of the segmentation septum, i.e. laterally *between* the metameric dorsal branches of the aorta (Fig. 6-7). The primordial intervertebral

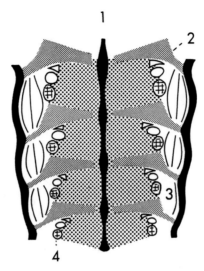

Figure 6-7. Diagram of a longitudinal section through the notochord *(1)* of a 7.5 mm embryo (Blechschmidt), stage 16, beginning of the 6th week (Carnegie no. 10309). Intervertebral disc zone is densely stippled *(2)*. Area of vertebral bodies is coarsely stippled. Lateral to vertebral bodies are veins (triangles), arteries (ovals), spinal nerves *(4)* and myotomes *(3)*.

discs are relatively thick. By the sixth week (11 mm embryos) the rib and vertebral arch primordia are clearly distinguishable (Fig. 6-8). A rearrangement of the vertebral column primordia that has been described in some textbooks was never evident to the authors. Such descriptions do not appear to be based on sufficient material and exact observations.

The wedge shape that the somites exhibit is a characteristic constructive component of whole trunk development. During the period of somite formation the positional relationships are significant. The volume of the amniotic fluid increases. Simultaneously, there is a relative decrease in the volume of the fluid within the intra– and extraembryonic coelomic cavities which still communicate with each other. This finding may be important in the kinetic development of the lateral body wall. The increasing difference between the volume of the amniotic and coelomic fluids probably causes growth adduction of the lateral body wall.

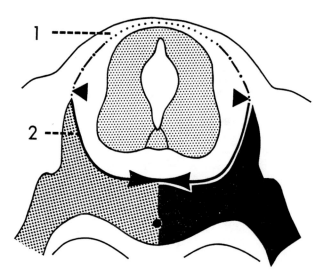

Figure 6-8. Diagram of a transversely cut section of an 11 mm embryo at the level of the thorax. The dorsal ectomeninx is still thin *(1)*, the ventral is thick *(2)*. Arrowheads represent the expansion pressure of the arachnoid fluid. Convergent arrows indicate the restraining function of the flattening part of the dura. On the right side is the precartilage of an intervertebral disc in solid black. The disc is continuous with a rib and with a neural process.

If this is the case, it would also contribute to the wedge shape of the developing somites.

The layer of tissue ventral to the somites and adjacent to the lining of the intraembryonic coelom (serosa) is of particular interest (Fig. 6-6). During its development it presents features that are characteristic of the very different developmental movements that occur in the dorsal and ventral body walls. Measurements taken of a series of stages show that the paired aortae shorten in relation to the neural tube. When the aortae shorten, they straighten and move together with the mesenteric root ventrally away from the convexly curved neural tube and notochord. Such a positional development does not occur in the region of the lateral wall of the embryonic coelomic cavity. Here, the lateral wall remains as the somatopleura that is attached dorsally in close contact with the ectoderm of the body wall. Because of its position, the intermediate tissue, forming the embryonic retrositus, rotates in the direction of the curved arrows in Figure 6-6. This developmental movement is fundamental to and characteristic of the excretory apparatus. As a result of its kinetic development the early excretory apparatus appears bilaterally as a longitudinal fold or bulge with cranial, intermediate and caudal segments. This fold may be understood as being a manifestation of the growth adduction of the lateral abdominal wall at the beginning of the second month. The topokinesis of this region will be described further in Chapter 11 with kidney formation.

7

LIMITING TISSUES AND INNER TISSUES

IF EXPERIMENTAL analyses alone could elucidate developmental relationships, then a knowledge of the morphology would be unnecessary. One would only have to conduct the experiments without any viewpoint and would then know what the requirements were, what occurs regularly and what the principles are that govern development. Unfortunately, experience has shown that this approach alone is inadequate and impractical. Morphological orientation is not only necessary for insights into where and under which circumstances experiments should be conducted, but also to reveal the various circumstances for obtaining a survey about differentiations and, as a result, to distinguish between important and unimportant facts. For example, a morphological knowledge of the body wall during embryonic development is necessary.

Near the end of the first month the embryo develops the following shape. Its length and circumference increase to such an extent that, relative to the umbilical area, the embryo projects dorsally and protrudes deeply into the amniotic cavity. During this period, the circumference of the umbilical area not only remains small but actually undergoes an absolute decrease. Because of this fact, the umbilical area is a good reference point when determining developmental movements of the embryo.

All partial differentiations that are distinguishable are consistent with, and are included in, the developmental dynamics of the whole embryo. If this assumption is correct, then not only are all the structures within the embryo important for differentiations to occur, but also their outer membranes and the extra-embryonic fluids.

There are no arteries demonstrable in the growing amnion of the early embryo. Yet, the total mass of the amnion increases. It must be concluded from this that nourishment of the amnion occurs by diffusion from the chorionic cavity that is immediately external to it. However, this movement would not exclude simultaneous metabolic movements from occurring in the opposite direction, i.e. metabolic water from the amniotic cavity passing into the chorionic cavity by way of the cytoplasm of the amnion cells.

The amniotic cavity develops from the lumen of the dorsal entoblast chamber. At the beginning of the second month, the fluid in this chamber (dorsal blastem fluid) quickly increases in volume at the expense of the preventral blastem fluid in the chorionic cavity. The dorsal blastem fluid is the anlage of the amniotic fluid. During this period, not only the yolk-sac mesoblast but also the chorionic mesoblast becomes progressively more vascularized. Because of this the diffusion of nutritive substances across the chorionic cavity probably loses its importance. In spite of this, transportation of nutrients towards the early embryo runs parathelially along the chorionic epithelium. At the same time, a movement appears to take place, namely, the resorption of more and more fluid from the chorionic cavity by the anlage of the placenta. The extremely thin amnion, which is hardly distinguishable with the naked eye, protrudes convexly towards the chorionic cavity. This protrusion is an indication of the pressure differences between the dorsal and preventral blastem fluids. It is reasonable to conclude that the stimulus for surface expansion of the amnion is the increased volume of the amniotic fluid.

The yolk sac retains its shape since its walls are thicker and it is richly vascularized. When the vascular meshes are filled with blood they cause the yolk-sac wall to arch convexly. By means of the vascularization, the circumference of the yolk sac increases locally at the vertex of its vascularized tissue meshes. From the development of the shape of the yolk sac, it becomes apparent that as the surface of the yolk sac enlarges distally by appositional growth, it simultaneously diminishes proximally (Fig. 7-1). Because of this, the yolk stalk (vitelline duct) collapses. It becomes thin as it lengthens and ruptures in approximately 6 mm embryos when the funnel-shaped umbilical cord sufficiently elongates. This occurs at the beginning of the second month. As the epithelial yolk stalk collapses and then ruptures, its stroma is stretched parallel to the long axis of the stalk. This occurs because of the extension produced by the growth of the wall of the umbilical coelom (arrows in Fig. 7-1). The stroma of the yolk stalk remains connected to the connective tissue of the midgut when the stalk ruptures. Because of this, the midgut is pulled by the yolk sac thus forming the umbilical loop (primary intestinal loop). This process prepares the way for herniation of the intestinal loop into the umbilical cord (1973, pp. 80 and 107). In the latter half of the second month, the umbilical hernia becomes particularly distinct since expansion of the liver is still slight, and consequently the abdomen is small during this period. Growth of the abdominal wall has not yet occurred as it is closely related to expansion of the liver since it has a position in front of the liver. The "reposition" of the coils of the herniated midgut into the abdominal cavity has not yet appeared. True repositioning of the intestinal coils caused by shortening of the coils is never observed.

There are other differentiations of the body wall during the second month that also appear to be functional processes and thus performances of the whole embryo. Dorsally, the surface ectoderm is expanded by the rapid eccentric growth of the brain and spinal cord. Ventrally, it is expanded by the heart and liver which enlarge by appositional growth and bulge near the ectoderm. As a result of the enlargement of the underlying structures, the dorsal and ventral body wall becomes thin (Figs. 7-2 and 7-4). The rapid

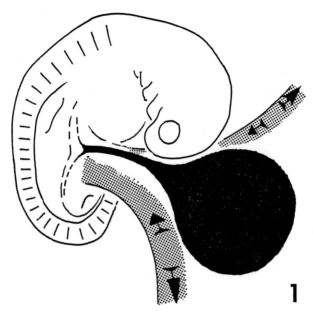

Figure 7-1. Drawing of a 4.2 mm embryo, five weeks. *1*, umbilical coelom. Arrows indicate growth movements in the region of the funnel-shaped anlage of the umbilical cord.

increase in surface area of these two regions causes them to exhibit remarkable kinetic features. Surface growth of the body wall between the dorsal and ventral regions is hindered. This causes the surface ectoderm in this zone to thicken and the underlying stroma to become dense. This region of the embryo is called the lateral field and is shown in lateral aspect (Fig. 7-2) and in a transverse section (Fig. 7-4). The locomotor apparatus and the very early peripheral nervous system make their first appearance in this field. The deep part of the field forms the axial skeleton. Dorsally the lateral field reaches to the central nervous system, and ventrally it is closely situated to the gut (Fig. 7-4).

Beneath the thin ectodermal cells, located dorsally and ventrally, the stroma is composed of mesenchymal meshes that have obtained a plate-like arrangement between the liquid intercellular substances (loose plate-like mesenchyma = Plattenmesenchym).

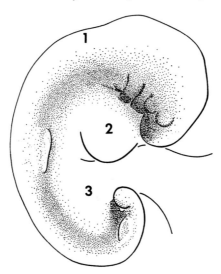

Figure 7-2. Lateral surface of a 4.2 mm embryo showing the position of thickened ectoderm (stipple) which forms a ring between the thin ectodermal dorsal *(1)* and ventral *(2* and *3)* body walls; Abdominal wall *(3)* more flattened than that in the heart area *(2).*

As the mesenchymal cells flatten they probably release substances into the interstices of the stroma. Regional comparisons consistently show that plate-like mesenchyma becomes loose as a result of fluid accumulating in the cell interstices. The fluid does not stagnate in the intercellular spaces. In the region shown in Figure 7-3, it partly flows from ventral to dorsalwards as the brain and the ventral body wall bend. In the body region shown in Figure 7-4, the plate-like mesenchyma is in a different situation. Dorsally, the fluid partly could arise from the neural tube and ventrally, from the intestines which are surrounded by the coelomic cavity. The thin, membrane-like dorsal and ventral body walls protrude or arch dorsally and ventrally, respectively. It is concluded from this that a pressure difference exists between the two sides of these walls with a higher fluid pressure on their inner aspect (Fig. 7-4, arrowheads). As a consequence of this pressure difference, fluid probably leaves the embryo and passes into the amniotic cavity. In contrast, the stroma deep to the laterally thickened ectoderm does not appear to be capable of releasing osmotically active katabolites. The stroma is densely packed with cells that are closely attached to each other, and the interstices in these regions contain little fluid. This anlage of the embryonic corium is already evident in these regions by the end of the first month (Fig. 7-3).

From the preceeding statements it becomes evident that the shape of the ectoderm which exhibits varying thicknesses is an

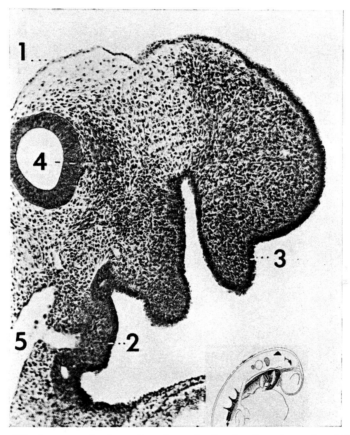

Figure 7-3. A parasagittal section through the head region of a 3.4 mm embryo, 27 somites, stage 12, approximately 27 days. 110×. *1*, thin ectoderm with delicate stroma; *2*, thick ectoderm with dense strong stroma (pharyngeal arch II); *3*, maxillary bulge; *4*, otic vesicle with neural crest of CN vii-viii); *5*, v. cardinalis sup. The diagram shows the biodynamics of the curving embryo as shown in Figure 8-3.

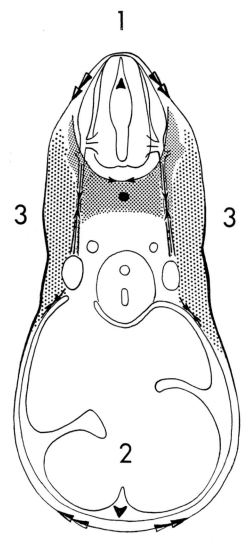

Figure 7-4. Transverse section through the heart region of an 8 mm embryo, stage 16, middle of 6th week. Dorsally over the spinal cord *(1)* and ventrally over the heart *(2)*, the epithelium is thin and the underlying stroma is loose. Between both, the epithelium of the lateral body wall is thickened, *(3)* and the underlying stroma is dense. Outlined, divergent arrows indicate regions of rapidly increasing surface area. Convergent arrows in the region of the ventral spinal nerve rami show their restraining function. Arrowheads represent fluid pressure.

instant expression of varying rates of growth. The growth rate is directly related to growth resistances that differ from one region to another. The resistances are types of extragenetic information for differentiations. Regional comparisons of the movements during development led to the formulation of the following principle. *Wherever ectoderm has the opportunity to expand because of its position and immediate occasion from the kinetic circumstances, it becomes relatively thin; when it is hindered in surface growth because of its position, it becomes relatively thick.* This phenomenon is comparable to the type of buildings constructed on any given plot of land. If a building site is cramped, the tendency is to build high-rise structures, perpendicular to the ground. Thick epithelium is comparable to this with its high and multiple layers of cells. On the other hand, when space is abundant, single-story buildings are constructed comparable to epithelium that has the occasion to expand rapidly, flatten, and in some areas, remain one cell thick. It is typical for such cells and their nuclei to become flattened. This principle supports the rule that cell shape is not determined from within itself but corresponds directly or indirectly to the position and shape of its neighboring structures. The shape of every organ or organism is not an inherent independent property of each structure. In general, shape is dependent on surrounding structures and is continuously adapting in a biodynamic way.

The thickened ectoderm on the right and left lateral body wall is continuous cranially in the (ventral) neck region and caudally in the region of the external genitalia. Since the area of ectodermal thickening has a circular configuration when viewed bilaterally, it is referred to as the *ectoderm ring* (Fig. 7-2). The whole formation, including its dense underlying stroma, forms a ring-shaped area of the body wall around the umbilical area; its distance from the umbilical area is greater cranially than caudally. The lateral portions of the ring have been interpreted previously from comparative anatomical studies as the milk or mammary ridges. However, the ridges are also evident in reptilian embryos where milk glands never develop. Because of this, such an interpretation falls short of being a constructive principle for understanding its formation.

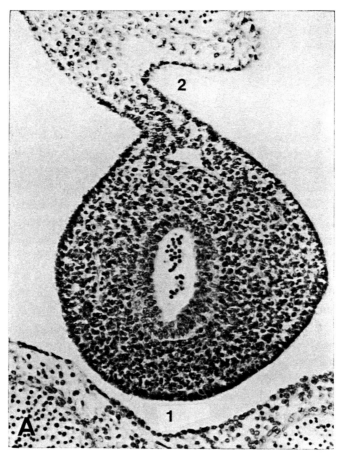

Figure 7-5 A and B. (*A*) Transverse section through the colon anlage of an 8 mm embryo. 180×. The longitudinal axis of the colon is bent in a con-cave manner ventrally. Below the intestinal anlage the ventral abdominal wall (*1*) contains blood-filled umbilical arteries. Above the anlage is the me-sentery (*2*) where the thickened visceral serosa is continuous with the thin parietal serosa. Beneath the thick epithelium the stroma has become dense.

Regional comparisons consistently show that the stroma that lies adjacent to thickened ectoderm exhibits intense blood vessel formation. As the ectoderm thickens, the number of its cells increases. The intense development of vessels in the underlying stroma is a consequence of ectoderm thickening. Under comparable circumstances, capillary formation is always greater near thick limiting tissue (ectoderm) than it is near thin limiting tissue. An example of this phenomenon is the rich blood supply located deep to the palm and sole where the ectoderm is very thick. Not only is the blood supply to these areas abundant in the adult, it is also discernible prenatally. The skin of these areas has a reddish coloration when compared to the pale-blue color of the thinner skin on the dorsum of the hand and foot. These observations support the statement that thick, limiting tissue with its closely arranged cells causes an increase in the metabolism of the underlying stroma with the metabolic intensity in a gradient toward the epithelium. In other words, in vivo metabolic movements that exhibit spatial order are brought about as a result of a prior differentiation or predevelopment. In regard to the early formation of capillaries, such metabolic movements are another application of the kinetic principle that states that *differentiations occur as being outside-inside differentiations*. Such outer differentiations initiate a determination which is a real limitation on developmental capacities. In more general terms this means that determinations depend on outer limitations whereas stability exists in the interior.

Another example of how developmental movements caused by surface growth in one region can be compared with those in another region is the limiting tissue of the embryonic serosa. The serosa is a surface layer on the interior of the embryo which expands differently in different locations. In the second month the parietal serosa in the abdominal region is expanded more than the visceral serosa on the intestinal anlage (Fig. 7-5). By comparing the two areas it becomes evident that the surface expansion of the parietal serosa is greater than that of the intestinal visceral serosa during this developmental period. As expected,

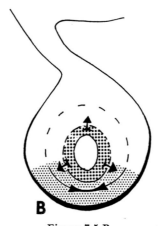

B

Figure 7-5 B.
(*B*) The diagram of the colon anlage shows its biokinetic features. Divergent arrows represent the expansion growth of the endoderm. Growth resistance of the stroma is indicated by convergent arrows.

the serosal epithelium of the tiny embryonic gut with its retarded surface growth is thick, and its underlying stroma is dense and highly vascularized. In the transitional zone between the gut and the dorsal abdominal wall (region of the developing mesentery), the thick epithelium of the intestinal visceral serosa is continuous with the thin epithelium of the parietal serosa and, at the same time, the underlying dense stroma is continuous with loose stroma.

From the functional standpoint, the main purpose of epithelia has been stated to be one of protection. There is no objective proof for such a statement. In fact, many body parts which are very exposed have an extremely thin epithelial covering and accordingly they are not protected very well. For example, in embryos the epithelium of the unprotected extensor side of the arm is extremely thin, but that of the sheltered axilla is thick. In truth, the thickness of epithelia is dependent on their position.

In many areas of the embryo, there are relatively large vascular spaces filled with blood in the vicinity of the epithelial surfaces. The importance of the pulsations of these spaces to surface growth has not yet been systematically investigated.

8

BLOOD VESSELS

BASED ON WHAT HAS BEEN SAID to this point, it now becomes possible to understand the manner in which blood vessels develop. Like all formations, blood vessels must first have a pre-development or prerequisite before they can make their appearance. Once this occurs there must then be adequate space at the proper moment in time, i.e. the immediate kinetic occasion.

Even if no other differentiations were investigated, the information on vascular development alone should be sufficient for one to realize that the common belief that differentiations possibly begin from within (in the sense of self-differentiation) is unsound. Never has an artery or vein been demonstrated to develop its in vivo branches in tissue culture. The origin of the paths for blood circulation cannot be described in any logical sequence without knowing the movements the circulatory paths undergo during development. In other words, it would be impossible for circulatory paths to begin in a living, developing organism without there simultaneously existing a developmental dynamics for the paths.

The topokinetics (kinetics of positional development) for blood vessel formation can be shown to be part of and consistent with the entire differentiation process. After comparing regions of the inner tissue immediately before and after the development of vascular paths, it becomes clear that they consistently form in zones that are bound into a three-sided configuration by other structures. These regions are called *canalization zones,* because they appear to be the predevelopment for the vascularization process. An example of a canalization zone can be seen in a 2.57 mm embryo (Fig. 8-1). This three-sided zone is bound by the ectoderm, neural tube and endoderm, respectively. It provides the space for the development of the first large artery anlage (dorsal aorta) on each side of the embryo (Fig. 8-2). The canalization zones can be demonstrated *before* the vessels are visible. The intercellular fluid in these zones prepares the way for the blood vessels. This is an important principle that veins, as well as arteries, appear to follow during their formation. Early veins arise from the coalescing of fluid vacuoles that form in intercellular spaces. Early arteries give rise to endothelial sprouts that grow into the cell interstices. Whether arteries or veins develop in the

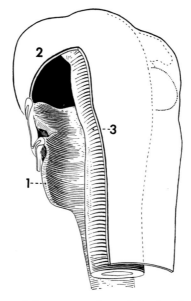

Figure 8-1. Part of a serial reconstruction of the head region of a 2.57 mm embryo, stage 12, 23 somites, approximately 26 days (Blechschmidt Collection, Carnegie no. 10305) showing the canalization zone between the endoderm (*1*), ectoderm (*2*) and neural tube (*3*).

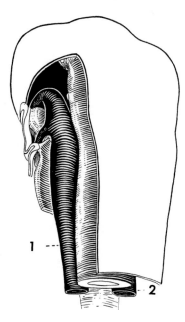

Figure 8-2. The same serial reconstruction as shown in Figure 8-1 with the left (*1*) and right (*2*) dorsal aortae in position. The dorsal aortae at this stage appear as long capillaries in the canalization zones.

canalization zone is evidently a result of the local metabolic gradient, i.e. the need for nourishment in a prior developed field and its positional relationship to the nutritional source.

After a blood vessel has grown sufficiently in any inner tissue, it then appears to have a *restraining function* (Haltefunktion) on the structures it supplies. The following occurs without exception: The longitudinal growth of each vessel stem is retarded when compared to the total length of its numerous branches. In this manner blood vessels have the capacity to cause a growth resistance that is directed against the organs they supply. This is another example of an important formative function that has never been described previously as a principle. As blood passes distalwards into the frequently branched capillaries it flows slowly as compared to its rate of flow in the more proximal vessel stems. Consequently, nearly all of the nutritive substances in the blood are able to pass through (permeate) the vascular wall distally and thereby leave the blood stream. Proximally, however, nutritive substances move faster along the wall of larger vessels. They do not leave the vessel but instead move along the endothelium (parmeate). The growth rate of this segment of vessels is therefore comparatively slow. The retarded lengthening of the vascular stems manifests itself as a restraining function in respect to more intensely growing tissues that have profuse capillaries.

Therefore, it is concluded from Blechschmidt's investigations that the increased bending of the embryo during the fourth and fifth weeks is very probably strictly correlated to the restraining function of the embryonic dorsal aortae. The convergent arrows in Figure 8-3 represent this restraining function and its resultant pulling effect on the cranial end of the embryo. In addition to the restraining function of the dorsal aortae, the lengthening of the neural tube appears also to play a role in the bending of the growing embryo. Since the nervous and vascular systems are connected

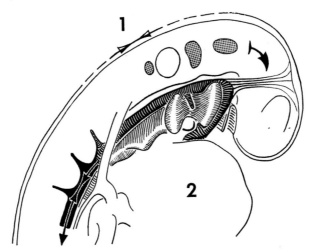

Figure 8-3. The cranial end of a serial reconstruction of the same embryo in Figure 8-1 (cf. 1973, p. 17). The restraining function of the dorsal aorta against the longitudinal growth of the neural tube is represented by converging arrows ventral to the neural tube. Lower arrow shows the growth pull of the right aorta. Bending of the neural tube (cephalic flexure) is shown by a curved arrow. Convergent arrows dorsal to the neural tube show the delicate, two-dimensional resistance of the ectoderm (*1*) on the dorsal surface of the embryo. *2*, heart.

by tissue, the brain appears to be bridled by the relative shortening of the dorsal aortae that lie close to the neural tube. As soon as the aortae bridle the ventral aspect of the expanding brain, the brain bends in a concave manner over the heart which is very large in this period. The position of the bending is in accordance with the position of the aortic bridle. As the bending occurs, the ectoderm and endoderm on the ventral side of the embryonic head and neck regions undergo characteristic foldings thereby establishing the arching folds (pharyngeal arches) (Fig. 10-1). In addition, this formation of outer shape is a measure of the formation of inner, related structures. This discovery will be explained in Chapter 10.

It is important to remember that the vascular system always contributes to the construction of subsequent formations because of the capabilities it developed in its own metabolic field. Blood vessels appear to be especially capable of acting as restrainers. Their restraining function not only pertains to the development of outer organs, e.g. body wall organs, but also to inner organs, e.g. the entire intestinal tract. One example among many is the development of the thyroid gland which can be explained in light of its relationship to the early formation of the aortae. By examining the early positional relationships of the aortae in a 2.5 mm embryo one observes the following (Fig. 8-4): The first pharyngeal arch artery (first aortic arch) on each side connects the unpaired ventral aorta (outflow of heart) with its corresponding dorsal aorta. Each first capillary arch artery forms an obtuse angle with its counterpart on the other side at their origin from the ventral aorta. This angle becomes progressively more acute as the heart, ventral aorta and other viscera move caudally (descent of viscera, *see* Chapter 10). The adjacent endoderm in the floor of the pharynx is gathered as the angle decreases thereby forming the unpaired anlage of the thyroid gland.

The epithelial anlage of the thyroid gland is connected by inner tissue to the foregut and the caudally migrating heart. Because of this, it subsequently loses its epithelial attachment to the pharyngeal endoderm as the heart migrates. The thyroid gland then becomes ductless, i.e. an endocrine gland. During their forma-

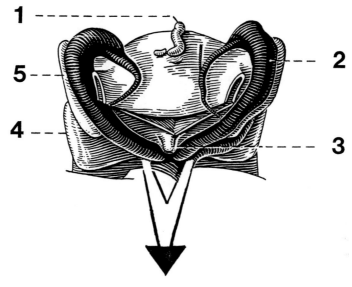

Figure 8-4. Head region (ventral aspect) of a 2.57 mm embryo showing the vascular relations of the arteries to the endoderm (vascular cage of aortae) (cf. 1973, p. 26). Arrow shows the direction of movement (descent) of the heart and ventral aorta. The angle between the diverging stems of the arrow indicates the angle that the first pharyngeal arch arteries (2) make with each other at their junction with the ventral aorta. When this angle becomes more acute as the heart and ventral aorta move caudally, the endoderm of the pharyngeal floor is gathered to form the epithelial anlage of the thyroid gland (3). 1, notochord; 4, second pharyngeal pouch; 5, first pharyngeal pouch.

tion endocrine glands lose their connection with the epithelium from which they arise. This is generally brought about as a result of their development kinetics. The chemical changes that accompany this are not yet known. Such information would be very helpful in understanding the molecular biology of these glands.

The developmental kinetics of ductless glands can be better understood by yet another example. The kinetics characteristic of such formations can be appreciated by comparing the position of the hypophysis and its surrounding structures at different stages of development. The increased bending of the embryo causes the brain to tilt more and more ventralwards. As this occurs the ectoderm in the roof of the stomodeum is compressed against the underside of the diencephalon and rolls upon itself, thereby forming the anlage of the orohypophysis (Rathke's pouch) (Fig. 8-5). The movement of Rathke's pouch is comparable to the movement of a broad belt around a wheel. During this rolling process, the orohypophyseal anlage loses its connection with its matrix epithelium (oral epithelium) and becomes ductless. In the period when the embryo becomes progressively curved and the hypophyseal duct lengthens, the mesenchyma that forms the common bed of the diencephalon and orohypophysis becomes stretched, forming the mesenchymal sella turcica (*see* convergent arrows in Fig. 8-6). As the mentioned mesenchymal tissue is stretched, it appears to exert a growth pull on the diencephalon immediately above the anlage of the orohypophysis (Fig. 8-6). The pull of the tissue of the wall of the diencephalon apparently causes the formation of a brain appendage, the anlage of the neurohypophysis. This positional development of the neurohypophysis initiates the known neurosecretory mechanisms.

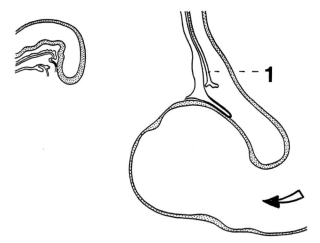

Figure 8-5. Midline relationships of the hypophyseal (Rathke's) pouch in 2.57 mm and 6.3 mm embryos. Development of the orohypophysis is biokinetically correlated with movement of growing brain (arrow). As the brain bends progressively, the pouch which is closely attached to the brain grows rapidly in length. *1*, notochord.

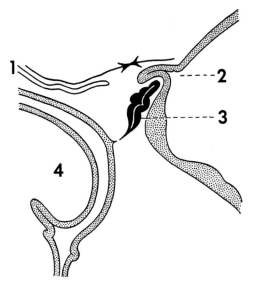

Figure 8-6. Midline relationships of the orohypophysis (*3*) in a 17.5 mm embryo. Convergent arrows indicate the restraining function of the mesenchyma in the area where the sella turcica arises. *1*, notochord; *2*, neurohypophysis; *4*, tongue.

9

NERVOUS SYSTEM

T HE TOTAL NERVOUS SYSTEM is fundamentally important for the differentiation of man. This importance is due not only to the cerebralization but also to the early development of the entire nervous system (neuralization).

POSITION AND SHAPE OF THE EMBRYONIC NERVOUS SYSTEM

After the first month the neural tube in the trunk region of the embryo can be recognized as the spinal cord and the enlarged cranial segment in the broad predeveloped head region is evident as the embryonic brain. The spinal cord is anchored in the trunk by numerous spinal nerves. Only a few cranial nerves course from the brain to the face, which is still relatively small. The brain is enclosed in tissue that will form the wall of the cranial cavity. Because of this enclosure the brain is hindered in longitudinal growth and consequently bends upon itself as it grows. At its frontal end it exhibits two blind-sac expansions on each side which are the anlagen of the optic cup and cerebral hemisphere (optic and cerebral vesicles) (Fig. 9-1).

Surface growth of the embryonic brain was mentioned in preceding chapters. At this time, it is important to point out that the dorsal side of the brain exhibits low resistance to growth. The

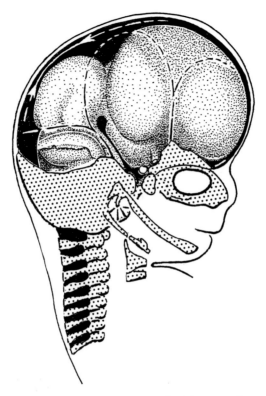

Figure 9-1. Preparation of the head region of a 29 mm embryo, stage 29, end of eighth week. Chondrocranium is shown as sparse stipple. The primitive arachnoid occupies the solid black areas. The arching interrupted lines show the position of the meningeal stretches (dural bands or girdles). Converging white arrows represent the low growth resistance in the pia mater anlage (cf., 1973, pp. 106, 112).

body wall in this area becomes easily expanded over the growing brain *(see* broken lines and converging arrows in Figs. 8-3 and 9-1). As a result of this the mesenchyma adjacent to the vertex of the brain becomes extremely flattened in the second month and is stretched to such a degree that its surface growth is retarded. The retarded growth of flattened tissue causes the antibasal portion of the cerebral hemispheres and metencephalon (anlage of cerebellar hemispheres) to remain close together. This positional development is an important predevelopment of the future proportions of the brain. Its subdivisions are understandable in light of the close connection of these two brain areas. The cerebral hemispheres grow dorsally and bend convexly above the eye and laterally over the outer aspect of the brainstem (Fig. 9-1).

Because of the manner in which the cerebral hemispheres grow during the second and subsequent months, the mesenchyma related to their expanding surfaces becomes biomechanically compressed and flattened. This occurs in the area between the cerebral hemispheres and between the hemispheres and the antibasal part of the transversely aligned cerebellum (rhombic lips). The compressed mesenchyma forms the falx cerebri between the cerebral hemispheres (Fig. 9-2). The tentorium cerebelli arises

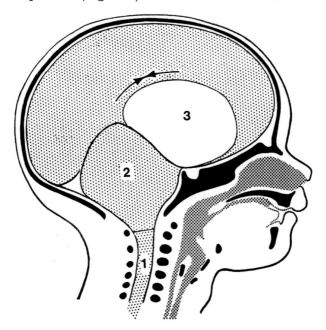

Figure 9-2. Drawing of the newborn head (after Hochstetter, 1946). Convergent arrows in area of fine, sparse stipple represent area of stretched mesenchyma between the cerebral hemispheres from which the falx cerebri is formed. *1*, dura mater of spinal cord; *2*, tentorium cerebelli that developed from the early stretched mesenchyma between the parietal lobe of the cerebrum and the cerebellum. Communication between right and left sides of cranial cavity is shown at *3*.

from the compressed mesenchyma between the cerebral hemi-spheres and the rhombic lips (cerebellum). These new findings reveal that position, shape and structure, as well as their changes, are features which relate to each other spatially and kinetically. Any one of these features for any given formation should never be considered separately and isolated from the others. As a result of these relationships it should be expected that the complexly con-structed nervous system also has relatively simple features which follow rules that are similar to those known for inanimate objects.

EARLY STRUCTURE OF THE EMBRYONIC
NERVOUS SYSTEM

At the beginning of the second month, the epithelium of the early neural tube has become thick and crowded with cells. The outer side of the epithelium is relatively fixed to the primitive meninx (anlage of the pia mater) but the inner side that is in contact with the fluid in the neurocoele is free. The numerous slender cell processes are peripherally arranged in a palisade in the wall of the neural tube. These peripheral parts of the cells that are adjacent to the pia mater anlage are so close to one another that there is no room for cell nuclei (Figs. 9-3 and 9-4). This outer (photographically) light zone will give rise to the white matter of the neural tube (marginal layer). The cell nuclei ac-cumulate in the inner, and therefore (photographically) dark, zone near the neurocoele where numerous ventricular mitoses occur (ependymal layer). If one interprets the zones of the em-bryonic neural tube as different metabolic fields, then the outer zone is near the source of nourishment and must therefore be con-sidered as an assimilation field. Likewise, the inner zone which is seen in sections to be (photographically) dark must be consid-ered as a dissimilation (katabolic) field.[7] Between the two totally different zones there exists an intermediate (photographically) grey zone that is composed of both cell nuclei and processes. The

---

[7]The authors have no argument for the possible assumption that the many large substances needed for the construction of cells are assimilated primarily from the neurocoele and that the smaller molecules, e.g. water, which are the products of dissimilation (katabolism), are released into the primitive meninx at the periphery.

nuclei are at central-peripheral positions to one another whereas the processes are in juxtaposition (Fig. 9-3). In other words, the embryonic wall of both the spinal cord and brain segments of the neural tube typically exhibit three zones. These zones are: (a) an *inner* zone containing a relatively large amount of liquid and adjacent to the neurocoele fluid, (b) an *outer* zone almost free of cell bodies and nuclei and composed of very narrow cell processes that are juxtaposed and perpendicularly aligned to the primitive pia mater and (c) an *intermediate* zone that contains cell processes as well as the cell bodies of long, spindle-shaped cells (Fig. 9-3, *1,2,3*). From the biokinetic viewpoint, the more liquid inner layer allows a considerable degree of nuclear mobility which leads to its high mitotic rate.

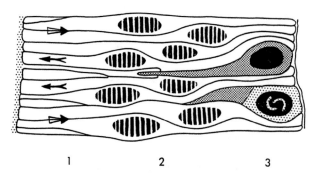

Figure 9-3. Diagram of the neural epithelium at the beginning of the second month. *1*, white zone (marginal layer); *2*, grey zone (mantle layer); *3*, black zone (ependymal layer). Stipple at left margin represents the anlage of the pia mater (primitive meninx). Arrows represent different movements that occur in the cytoplasm and the cell limiting membranes, respectively.

It is apparent from the cell arrangement that the cell limiting membranes, which are perpendicular to the limiting surfaces of the neural tube, have an alignment that is characteristic of a trajectory. The position, shape and structure of the three different zones of the central nervous system must be considered together when regarding the growth functions of these zones. With such an understanding, it is then possible to describe conclusively their kinetics during development.

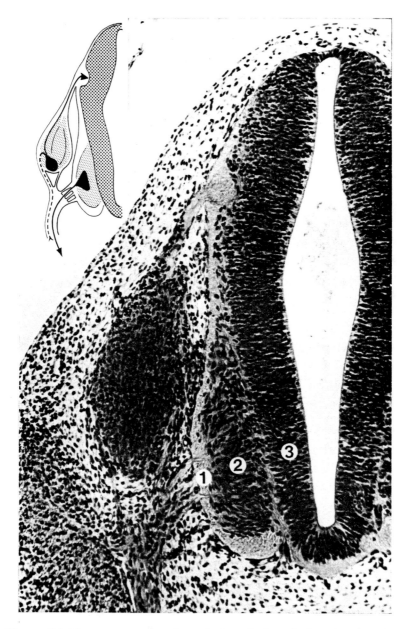

Figures 9-4. Transverse section through the spinal cord of an 8 mm embryo, stage 16, sixth week, 140×. (Blechschmidt Collection). *1,* white zone (marginal layer); *2,* grey zone (mantle layer); *3,* black zone (ependymal layer). Diagram at upper left shows the developmental movements of a spinal nerve in the region of its roots. Arrows indicate fluxion directions of establishing afferent and efferent nerve fibers.

Regional comparisons of the movements of the nervous system anlage during development show that its growth rates are related to its position and are therefore different from one locus to another. Dorsally, where the body wall is thin, there is little resistance to neural tube growth. There are only thin, plate-like mesenchymal cells under the very thin ectoderm in this region (Fig. 9-4). The fluid from the metabolic field of the neural tube flows into the interstices of the mesenchyma. The number of (ventricular) mitoses in the ependymal layer is greater dorsally than it is ventrally. This indicates that the dorsal part of the central nervous system grows appositionally. The cells have better access to space at the free surface of the embryo. Layering of the tube is initially absent in this region. In other words, the entire central nervous system of early and late embryos shows a marked increase in circumference dorsally. During this period its ventral portion (region of the floor plate) hardly grows at all.

When considered in three dimensions, these unequal developmental movements contribute to the kyphotic-like bending of the embryo. As the neural tube undergoes dorsal appositional growth, the mesenchyma (primitive meninx or embryonic dura) relatively soon becomes thickened ventrally more than dorsally (Fig. 9-5, heavy black line). This is already evident by the time the somites first appear. New cells that form in the neural tube wall must wedge in between previously formed cells. Consequently, the growth pressure of the neural tube increases, especially ventrally where the primitive meninx is tight. The primitive meninx in this region becomes extremely stretched against the expanding neural tube and the fluid that is produced by it. In this manner, the primitive meninx becomes resistant to tension and so strong in the embryo that it is possible to isolate it by dissection and actually tear it with forceps. In situ, this stretched mesenchyma acts as a restraining apparatus (Halteapparat) (Fig. 9-5, converging white arrows in right diagram). The growth pull of this primitive dura acts tangentially on the dorsal part of the neural tube thereby initiating the formation of neural crests which subsequently give rise to the large sensory ganglia and the dorsal roots that are located dorsally on each side (Fig. 9-5, left diagram). During the period when the primitive meninx exerts this forming function, it is supported in the trunk region by the dorsal intersegmental branches of the aorta, because these vessels remain short and are anchored in the primitive meninx by way of their branches. In the head region the pulling function that the meninx exhibits is assisted by the growth retardation of the pharyngeal arch vessels.

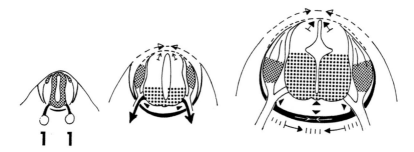

Figure 9-5. Cross-sectional diagrams of spinal cords in embryos approximately 3 mm, 7 mm and 8 mm (left to right) showing developmental movements of the spinal cord and ectomeninx. *1*, intersegmental branches of the dorsal aortae. Thick arrows represent growth pull of the spinal nerves. Arrows with base lines indicate the growth expansion of the spinal cord. Dorsal convergent arrows show growth resistance in the surface of the early cutis. White arrows show the restraining function of the ventral ectomeninx. Convergent arrows with base lines indicate the mesenchymal densation in the region of establishing vertebral column. Arrowheads represent fluid pressure in the arachnoid.

DORSAL AND VENTRAL ROOTS

Neural crests are cell aggregations that appear to be tangentially pulled from the dorsolateral side of the neural tube. These aggregations exist only dorsolaterally and move tangentially away from the central nervous system. This cell movement can be explained entirely by the kinetics of the surrounding structures (that are as follows). The neural tube grows intensely in the dorsal direction. The primitive meninx initially becomes strong in its ventral part. As the neural tube grows, the neural crest cells are pulled out of the neural tube by the tensile strength of the meninx and the restraining function of the dorsal intersegmental vessels. A so-called "migration" of crest cells from the neural tube, as though they are driven by an inner impulse, has never been demonstrated nor should it be expected. The apparent biomechanical sliding of tissue is not truly mechanical but very much alive. It does not occur as an isolated local process but as a cooperative action with several partners, especially the neural tube, primitive meninx and blood vessels. Even in mathematics there are functions to which several partners would contribute. The concept of isolated solitary functions of developing structures is absurd.

It is important to note that the sliding process mentioned above occurs in the early grey matter of the dorsal portion of the neural tube. It is because of this sliding that the well-known butterfly configuration can be observed later in transverse sections of the spinal cord. Then the dorsal (posterior) horn of the grey matter appears only as a small appendage of the large and broad ventral (anterior) horn, the cells of which have not migrated from the neural tube. The primitive meninx restrains the ventral part of the neural tube so severely that the ventral median fissure forms when growth of the floor plate becomes retarded (compare Figs. 9-4, 9-10, 13-1, 13-2).

In the floor-plate region, the cell nuclei near the neurocoele lack sufficient space to divide. They then move towards the periphery. However, the cytoplasm in this region of the neural tube has been compressed and appears to be reduced in water content. Such conditions would not be favorable for mitosis. The initiation of retarded growth of the floor of the neural groove was described in Chapter 4 as a constructive factor during the formation of the axial process. As the above developmental movements take place, the ventral part of the primitive dura mater becomes so strong that fluid is congested between the dura mater and pia mater. The fluid appears to be pressed out of the neural tube through the interstices of the endomeninx (pia mater anlage) and is the anlage of the arachnoid fluid (Fig. 9-5, arrowheads). This accumulation of fluid forms the first cisterns of the embryonic arachnoid, i.e. on the ventral aspect of the spinal cord and on the basal aspect of the brain, particularly at the mesencephalon.

The fluid-filled meshes of arachnoid spaces enlarge and form a cushion along the growing neural tube. This is another example of accumulated fluid exhibiting biomechanical expansion forces. Such accumulations functionally contribute to differentiations. The authors' preparations consistently show that the fluid cushion expands only as far as the zone where the ventral roots arise. The expanding fluid appears to push the ventral end of the spinal ganglia laterally. This lateral displacement would then bring about a growth pull between the ventral end of the spinal ganglia and the spinal cord. It is in this area that the ventral roots arise perpendicular to the spinal cord surface. Ventral root formation seems to be a yielding of the spinal cord to this growth pull (Figs. 9-4 and 9-5). It would be impossible for the large cell bodies to become displaced out of the spinal cord zone where the ventral roots originate. In order to become displaced they would have to move through the minute interstices in the meshwork of the endomeninx that has become very vascular at the assimilation surface of the spinal cord.

At this time the neurocoele becomes rhomboid-shaped on transverse section. This shape change can be explained by the growth pull of the ventral roots (Fig. 9-4). The lateral tilting of the forms when growth of the floor plate becomes retarded (compare basal plate occurs as an early constructive function of the strong ventral roots between the spinal cord and the point where they branch. When consideration is given to the shape of the basal plate at different periods it is apparent that the plate gradually becomes thicker as development proceeds. Consideration of the associated change in cell structure reveals that there is not only a gradual increase in cell number but also the formation of progressively larger cells. Many of the cells form the large ventral horn cells which become the known motor centers. Their formation is typical of how the nucleo-cytoplasmic relationship changes. The large bodies of the ventral horn cells result from the formation of the ventral root fibers and are not the cause of the latter. The nerve fiber pathways are determined by their positional relationships and the large cells of the grey matter are demonstrable only after nerve fibers have arisen.

Unfortunately, the common term "nucleo-cytoplasmic ratio"

implies the misleading concept that the formation of the cytoplasm is dependent on the nucleus. The authors believe the exact reverse of this to be true. The development of the position, shape and structure of the nucleus is influenced mainly by conditions that exist outside itself. From this viewpoint, the nucleo- cytoplasmic ratio would more accurately be expressed as the cytoplasmo-nuclear ratio. The latter term would emphasize that the direction of the processes which initiate differentiation is from outside to inside and not the reverse. Also in this regard, the chapter title "Centers and Pathways" commonly used in many textbooks should be written more properly in the reverse. It is clearer to emphasize first the formation of the pathways, then their resultant centers. This means that in regard to the ventral roots, bundles of nerve fibers in these roots grow longer and increase in number as peripheral organs grow (the number of nerve fibers is dependent on peripheral organ growth). As this occurs, the cell bodies and nuclei in the related centers enlarge. This enlargement *follows* rather than *precedes* the lengthening of the nerve fibers. The enlargement of the cells is in correlation with the immediately surrounding glial cells.

Since the kinetics of dorsal and ventral root formation is different, one should conclude that their associated functional development must also be different.

PERIPHERAL NERVES

From the biomechanical viewpoint, *nerves are structures which are pulled.* This conclusion is reached from the following observations. When an approximately 3 mm embryo is prepared it can be demonstrated that the relatively straight nerves are fixed at their point of origin as well as at their insertion point. Initially, all the nerves are aligned in the shortest connection between "origin" and "insertion" and are regularly narrowed into a "waist" shape (Fig. 9-9). This finding leads to the conclusion that the membranes of the nerve fibers are stressed by tension longitudinally and circularly. This assumption provides an explanation for the round cross section of the growing nerves.

An example of neural structures being differentiated by pull is the growing of the embryonic optic nerve (Fig. 9-6). When the brain expands the distance between "origin" and "insertion" of the optic nerve increases, and accordingly the optic nerve becomes pulled and lengthens. In the second month the optic nerve, after having been initially short and thick, becomes slender and elongated. The proportions of the nerves during development lend support to the concept that their spatial structure is brought about as a result of pulling forces. The tensile strength of nerves can be easily demonstrated with anatomical methods.

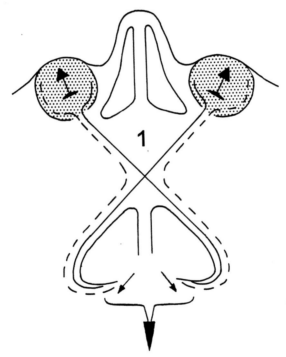

Figure 9-6. Diagram showing growth directions of the optic nerve fibers. Developmental movements of the eyeballs (top) in relation to the lateral geniculate nuclei (bottom) are indicated by arrows. *1*, optic chiasm.

Blechschmidt's collection of whole embryo serial reconstructions shows that cranial and spinal nerves as well as the sympa-

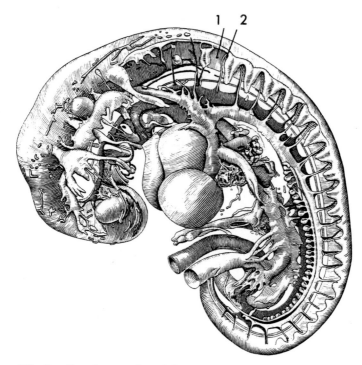

Figure 9-7. Details of a total serial reconstruction of a 4.2 mm embryo (Blechschmidt Collection) showing the relationship between the dorsal inter-segmental vessels (guiding structures) and the neural crest segments (spinal ganglion anlagen). Notice the greater distance between the neural crest segment and the succeeding dorsal intersegmental vessel *(1)* than between the vessel and the succeeding neural crest segment (*2*).

thetic trunk arise in close contact with blood vessels (Figs. 9-7 and 9-8). It was pointed out above that the neural crests appear to be pulled ventrally by the ventrally thickened primitive meninx which functions as a restrainer. As this occurs, the (intersegmental) blood vessels, dorsally near the spinal cord, seem to help cause displacement of the neural crest cells resulting in their subdivision into a serrated band on each side of the neural tube. The "teeth" (neural crest segments) in the band are the first manifestations of spinal ganglia and spinal nerves. They grow out of the spinal cord where the metameric capillary veins make contact with the

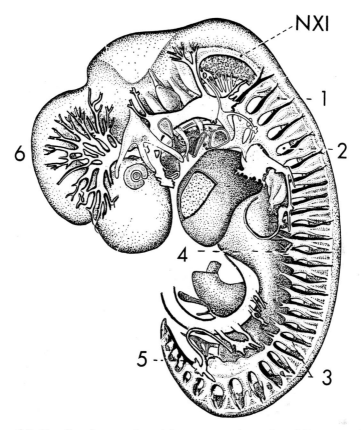

Figure 9-8. Details of a total serial reconstruction of a 7.5 mm embryo (Blechschmidt Collection) showing the relationship between the veins and the nerves. Notice that each dorsal intersegmental vein (black) is adjacent to the succeeding spinal ganglion (*1*) but there is a gap (*2*) between the spinal ganglion and the next succeeding dorsal intersegmental vein. The waist-like shape of the spinal nerves should be understood as resulting from growth pull. *3*, dorsal branches of the inferior (post) cardinal vein; *4*, dorsal border of peritoneum where the ventral ramus divides; *5*, inferior (post) cardinal vein; *6*, mesencephalon with anterior venous plexus.

capillary arteries. The number of spinal nerves corresponds exactly to the number of dorsal intersegmental tributaries of the cardinal veins. The cardinal vein tributaries that course from the spinal cord appear to exert the main pull on the spinal cord. It is precisely in these regions that the spinal nerves appear. The dorsal tributaries of the cardinal veins originate earlier than the spinal nerves (Figs. 9-7 and 9-8, lower trunk area). Subsequently, they appear to act as guiding structures for the nerves.

Also, in the head region the vascularization contributes to the localization of the cranial nerves. The latter become established in the head region as soon as paths of intercellular materials prepare the localization of blood vessels. When the brain nerves have sufficiently lengthened they use the stretched mesenchyma in the pharyngeal arches as a guiding structure. As an example, the reconstruction of a 4.2 mm embryo shows that all cranial and spinal nerves are related to blood vessels (Fig. 9-7). Spinal nerves are always closely attached to the veins. This attachment is a result of the ascent of the neural tube.

As the neural tube lengthens by growth, the distance increases between the spinal cord and the body wall veins at the dorsal border of the serosa. As a result, the tributaries of the cardinal veins exert a pull on the spinal ganglia. The spinal ganglia together with their dorsal roots become slender. When the embryo becomes erect the spinal nerves that previously converge towards one another in their ventral course subsequently align parallel to each other (compare Figs. 9-7, 9-8, 9-9). When the ventral ends of the spinal nerves spread apart, the distance between them quickly increases. The sudden increase in distance occurs along the mesonephric vein near the dorsal border of the serosa. The mesenchyma in these regions is stretched and becomes the guiding structure for the sympathetic trunk. Fibers of spinal nerves grow into the guiding structure thereby forming the sympathetic trunk.

Cartilage subsequently forms around the nerves and blood vessels. Since the nerve and vessel pathways are present by the second month, subsequent formation of the skeleton cannot occur in the space already occupied with these structures. Nerves and vessels are usually described as coursing through canals and foramina, for example, in the base of the skull. However, this description is misleading from the embryological viewpoint. As is known, the skeleton arises only after the nerve and blood vessel pathways have been established. From the developmental aspect,

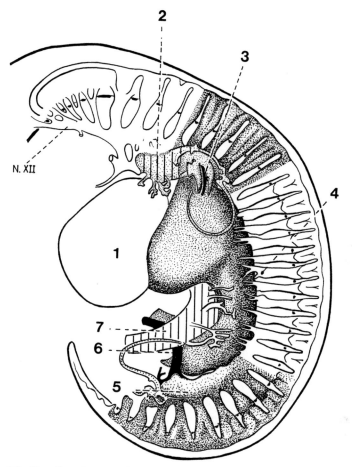

Figure 9-9. Details of a partial serial reconstruction of the same embryo shown in Figure 9-8 showing medial (communicating) ramus and lateral (ventral) ramus of the spinal nerve (*4*) at the dorsal border of the peritoneum. (cf. 1973, p. 57). *1*, heart; *2*, common cardinal vein; *3*, brachial artery; *5*, lumbosacral plexus; *6*, umbilical artery; *7*, umbilical vein.

it would be more accurate to say the skeleton surrounds the nerves and blood vessels.

The fundamental morphological connections of the peripheral nervous system and, consequently, its functional arrangement are developed by the beginning of the second month. Just as the shape of the head, cervical, trunk and limb regions differ so does the nerve circuitry differ in each of these regions. The spinal nerves in the trunk region exhibit the most regular arrangement. They course to the dorsal border of the peritoneum where they branch into nerves for the abdominal wall and the intestines. The spinal nerves in the region of the limb are also established in the second month. Their differentiation is determined decisively by the position and shape of the early cutis of the limbs. In the region of the limbs, the limb bud ectoderm, which is restricted in base expansion, brings the spinal nerves in contact with each other. In the region of the limb base, the contacting spinal nerves form the brachial and lumbosacral plexuses. In animals this interdependence has been demonstrated by experimental investigations.

CENTRAL PATHWAYS AND CENTERS

Processes of nerve cell bodies collectively form the so-called "white matter" that contains the system of central pathways. As the cell processes develop, the cell bodies, now sufficiently aggregated, form the grey matter that contains the system of centers or nuclear groups. Dorsal appositional growth of the neural tube causes the embryo to rapidly increase in its longitudinal and transverse diameters. As this growth occurs, the anlagen of the spinal ganglia are anchored ventrally by the strong, dense primitive meninx. Because of the anchoring, the distance increases between the dorsal zone of the neural tube and the spinal preganglia. In accordance with these developmental movements of the spinal ganglia, their contained cells send processes (neurites) into the guiding structure connecting the neural tube and the ganglia (diagram in Fig. 9-4). Because of the longitudinal growth of the early spinal cord, the processes of the spinal preganglion cells become the first ascending central pathways that are important for sensory conduction *(see* oval bundle in Fig. 9-4).

From the above finding alone, one could conclude that development of the central nervous system implies the simultaneous development of functioning afferent and efferent central pathways (tracts) and centers. Nothing has been found to support the idea that the function of the nervous system is added *after* the development of its shape and cell structure. It is the authors' opinion that function and structure develop simultaneously. The beginning of the nervous system implies the simultaneous beginning of function. The establishing functions are not identical to the definitive ones. Development of functions is also found in the nervous system. The functions physiologically investigated as being conductions are not the primary functions.

The development of the position, shape and structure of the early brain and spinal cord are morphological constructive actions. These actions are important for the total functional development of the embryo. In contrast to the brain, the spinal cord grows intensely in length in the relatively narrow vertebral canal. It becomes slender in comparison to the brain which becomes folded in its much broader area. As the embryonic spinal cord lengthens, the nerve anlagen remain anchored peripherally in the body wall. This is particularly true with the nerve anlagen in the caudal trunk region. On the basis of these movements, the white matter, which is lacking in cell bodies and nuclei, is structured in a longitudinal manner (Fig. 9-10). The tissue in this spinal cord zone slides particularly longitudinally along its surrounding tissue bed. These nerve pathways are established before their corresponding centers develop. In other words, the peripheral (outer) differentiation precedes the development of the centers.

Circularly aligned nerve fibers also arise when the neural tube grows in diameter. As the spinal cord enlarges eccentrically its more central layers slide in a dorsal direction against the more peripherally situated layers. The growing spinal cord "bursts" in a dorsal direction (arrows with base lines in Fig. 9-11). We believe that the U-shaped fiber paths arise as a result of the antagonistic growth movements of the ependyma against the outer layer *(see* U-shaped fibers and lines in Figs. 9-10 and 9-11, respectively). The summit of the U-shaped fibers forms the commissure in the floor plate of the spinal cord.

The cell limiting membranes in the developing spinal cord do not cross at any random angles but in regular planes perpendicu-

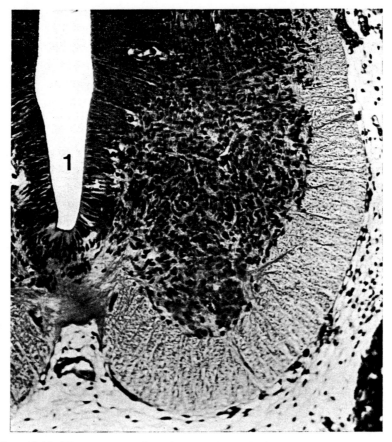

Figure 9-10. Transverse section through the spinal cord of a 19 mm embryo, stage 20, eighth week, 150× (Blechschmidt Collection) showing the trajectorial arrangement of cell limiting membranes. The ascending and descending fiber bundles are shown as small dots in the white matter. Compare with diagram in Fig. 9-11. *1,* central canal.

lar to one another. This feature is illustrated in Figure 9-11 by lines that form perpendiculars. These demonstrate that the developing spinal cord structure is arranged as a trajectory. The spatially ordered constructive functions of this development are prerequisites for ordered nervous system functions that appear later.

The cell limiting membranes of the embryonic brain also show particular growth directions which are favored biodynamically

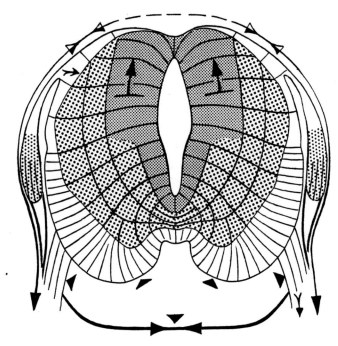

Figure 9-11. Cross-sectional diagram of the spinal cord of a 19 mm embryo showing the developmental movements and the alignment of the cell limiting membranes. Compare Fig. 9-10. Arrowheads represent fluid pressure between the endo– and ectomeninx. Tailed arrows in dorsal and ventral roots show flow movements consistent with the diagram in Figure 9-4. Other arrows are consistent with those shown in Figure 9-5.

(Fig. 9-12). One can demonstrate in the brain as well as in the spinal cord inner and outer limiting layers that are connected by a third zone. Photographically, these zones appear just as they do in the spinal cord, i.e. white, grey and black. Each zone is locally modified in accordance with the specific position and shape of the brain. Generally, however, the principles of dynamics for brain development are the same as those for spinal cord development.

As the embryonic brain grows eccentrically, the antibasal part of the cranial cavity wall yields to the growing brain by intense surface enlargement. In contrast, growth of the mesenchyma surrounding the growing brain is hindered basally. Consequently,

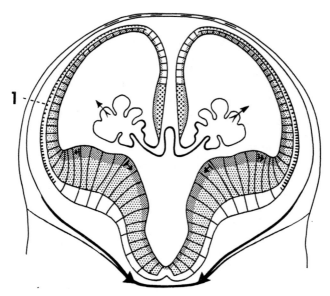

Figure 9-12. Diagram of a coronal section through the forebrain of a 27.2 mm embryo, stage 22, end of eighth week. Convergent arrows at base of brain represent growth resistance (restraining function) of the ectomeninx (anlage of dura mater) that is thickened in this area. The cerebral hemisphere wall is thin compared to the wall of the spinal cord (Fig. 9-11). The ventricles are large and contain fluid that arises from the choroid plexus (tailed arrows). Divergent arrows show the extensive growth and protrusion of the ventral grey where surface growth of the basal brain is locally hindered by the restraining function of the stretched ventral ectomeninx. *1,* superficial cell layer (cerebral cortex) separation of matrix by shearing.

the mesenchyma on its basal aspect (anlage of the dura mater) becomes very strong and resistant to tension (Fig. 9-12, convergent arrows). Once again mesenchymal tissue is encountered which becomes stretched during growth and functions as a restrainer in this instance against the brain. The brain adapts to this restraining function and consequently enlarges more and more eccentrically. The antibasal and dorsolateral parts of the cranial wall are thin and therefore present little resistance to the eccentric growth. However, the resistance to growth exerted by the cranial wall gradually increases more and more. When this occurs, large parts of the expanding brain fold against each other thereby forming the known, so-called "fissures." The falx cerebri and the tentorium cerebelli become stretched in the fissures. Some areas of the brain grow convexly in such a way that they gradually abut against one another. The ectomeninx (anlage of the dura mater) in the areas of abutment becomes stronger forming restraining bands or (dural) girdles (Fig. 9-1, interrupted arching lines). In the following months, only the surface of the brain between the bands grows intensely. The dural girdles (restraining bands) appear to curb brain growth to such a degree that the brain actually bulges the areas ("windows") between the bands. The clinically important fontanelles are established antibasally between the crescent-shaped borders of the bands. In other words the anlagen of the fontanelles become apparent before the osseous tissue of the skull is formed.

The intense thickening of the grey matter in the ventral part of the embryonic spinal cord was previously noted as a manifestation of the developmental dynamics of the growing spinal cord. Thickening of the ventral grey matter is even more evident in the embryonic cerebral hemispheres (cerebral vesicles) because their eccentric growth is more extensive. In the base of the developing hemispheres where surface growth is retarded, cells diverge toward the brain ventricle, i.e. in the direction of least resistance. The basal ganglia result from this brain wall thickening (Fig. 9-12, divergent arrows).

More is known today concerning the establishment of the cerebral cortex than was a few years ago. When the embryonic cortex is measured in a series of closely related stages, it becomes obvious that during cortical differentiation growth is not the same in each area. In the second month it is primarily the mantle layer of the embryonic cerebral hemispheres that expands. Here, the wedge-shaped "epithelial" cells of the cerebral wall are in close contact with the supplying stroma. With appositional growth of the antibasal areas (frontal and occipital portions) the circumference of the hemispheres rapidly increases. In the second month the lateral surface of the cerebral wall thereby becomes less curved or, in other words, flattens. Prior to the flattening the limiting membranes of the cortical cells exhibit an overall convergence inwards towards the ventricle. After the surface curvature is reduced, these cells become aligned more parallel to one another (Fig. 9-13). The establishing neurites of these cells become more and more straightened and establish the early embryonic pyramidal fibers. As the circumference of the brain increases by dorsal appositional growth the white matter exhibits a "fluxion field" for all descending neurites. The palisade-like peripheral cells enlarge more as the pyramidal fibers lengthen (nucleo-cytoplasmatic ratio) (Fig. 9-13). The establishment of the cortical grey matter is a result of the development of the pathways of the white matter (the so-called "nucleus semiovalis") which subdivides the cerebral wall forming an outer and an inner grey layer.

As the cerebral surface enlarges in three dimensions the cell processes also align in three dimensions, i.e. parallel as well as perpendicular to the anlage of the pia mater. The cell bodies have the greatest ability to enlarge in the area where cell processes intersect. The enlarged cells in the intersections frequently become spherical and many nuclei undergo mitoses (for more detailed illustrations, *see* 1961, p. 251).

It has become obvious that intense, eccentric, antibasal growth of the cerebral hemispheres is an important prerequisite for the high degree of differentiation of the human cortex.

The endomeninx (anlage of the pia mater) lies adjacent to the brain wall and contains many blood vessels. As the ventricle wall attempts to expand by each vascular pulsation, the thin weak areas of the hemispheres (medial walls) protrude in the direction of least resistance, i.e. toward the ventricles. These vascular protrusions become the choroid plexuses which release fluid into the ventricles (Fig. 9-12, tailed arrows). The chemical processes associated with this movement are still unknown.

GROWING NERVE FIBER TIPS

How do peripheral nerves find their way and attain their definitive arrangement? Just as it is with blood vessels in tissue culture (artificially isolated tissue), so it is with growing nerve fibers.

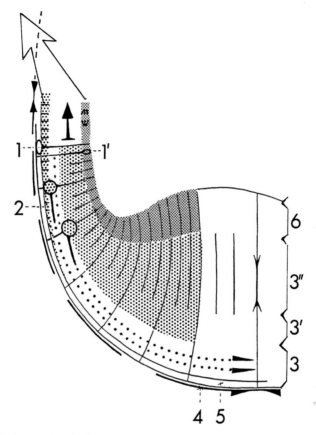

Figure 9-13. Details of Fig. 9-12. Segment of the brain wall of the 27.2 mm embryo is shown lateral to the basal ganglion. *1*, a cell from which the nucleus has migrated towards the surface of the brain (glial cell); *1'*, a cell with its nucleus lying next to the ventricular liquid (ependymal cell); *2*, cell-crowded zone of cerebral cortex; *3*, cerebral cortex formed by the marginal zone and the cell-crowded and fiber-crowded zones; *3'* and *3"*, loose and dense grey zones, respectively, (mantle layer) shown by sparse stipple; *4*, pia mater; *5*, marginal zone; *6*, black zone (ependymal layer) represented by dense stipple. Two circles represent neurons (ganglionic cells). Arrow with base line indicates the growth pressure of the cell bodies. Convergent arrows show the growth pull of cell limiting membranes and the pia mater. Arrowheads in zone *3* show growth direction of the neurons. The outlined arrow represents the growth movement of the cerebral wall.

In neither instance can normal branching occur. Normal developmental movements are required for a normal course or arrangement of both vessels and nerves. Blechschmidt's investigations indicate that normal pathways during development are guided in situ by previously formed structures. After they have formed, all such vascular and neural pathways act as restrainers. Regional comparisons of developmental movements reveal that both types of pathways require canalization as a prerequisite for finding their way. In the case of nerves these areas are referred to as "fluxion zones" rather than canalization zones (the term used in reference to blood vessel formation). The term "fluxion zones" implies that the direction in which nerve fibers grow is determined in fields where metabolic movements have a specific spatial order and present specific fluxion or flowing movements. A metabolic gradient would have to exist in such zones. Without such a gradient, flow would be impossible.

The branching area of the trigeminal nerve may be used as an example for the demonstration of a fluxion zone. The following information is the result of making exact comparisons of the morphology at different stages of early trigeminal nerve formation. The inner tissue (mesenchyma) in the early face region is not of the same thickness in each area of the face. In other words, the distance varies between the outer ectoderm and the brain and/or endoderm. This is the space occupied by mesenchyma. The mesenchymal tissue over the brain protrusions appears thin and relatively colorless (pale). The appearance of this tissue is comparable to the stretched tissue over a knuckle when the interphalangeal joint is strongly flexed. Mesenchymal tissue with this appearance is found over the embryonic cerebellum, mesencephalon and cerebrum (Fig. 9-14, *1,2,3*). It is also present lateral to the optic vesicle, lateral to the mouth *(4)* and at the embryonic eardrum *(5)*. In the areas between these thin fields of mesenchyma, the inner tissue is thick in the form of relatively large bands. These mesenchymal bands act as guiding structures for the three major branches of the trigeminal nerve, ophthalmic, maxillary and mandibular branches. The first band is located between the optic vesicle and the mesencephalon and acts as a guiding structure or path for the establishment of the ophthalmic nerve. The second band, between the optic vesicle and the mouth, is the guide for the establishment of the maxillary nerve. Between the mouth and the eardrum anlage of the middle ear one finds a third mesenchymal band that functions as the guiding structure for the origin of the mandibular nerve. All three areas of inner tissue thickening can be distinguished in 2 and 3 mm embryos *before* trigeminal nerve branches appear.

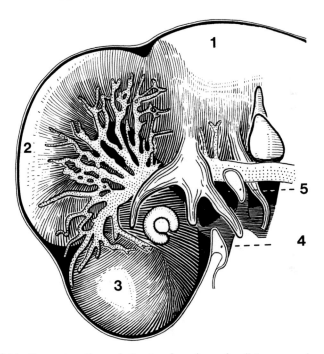

Figure 9-14. Reconstruction of the head region of a 7.5 mm embryo, stage 16, beginning of sixth week, showing position and relations of trigeminal nerve branches. *1, 2, 3,* areas of brain that are adjacent to the overlying ectoderm and without remarkable vascularization in the stroma; *4, 5,* areas of endoderm that are adjacent to the ectoderm (corner of mouth and eardrum).

Each of the thickened areas of mesenchyma is structurally characterized by collections of long, spindle-shaped cells. As a result of being compressed in narrow zones, this structure enables the intercellular substance to become aligned in these areas into minute canals that function as guiding paths for the small nerve fibers. The tiny, primary pathway for an ingrowing nerve fiber is consistently in an intercellular area between three neighboring, spindle-shaped, mesenchymal cells. Bundles of fibers are microscopically visible as nerves (Fig. 9-14).

It is important to keep in mind the principle that states that *before any new structure can begin there must first be adequate space and the immediate kinetic occasion.* Evidently the thick bands of mesenchyma provide the proper spatial opportunity for the establishment of the three trigeminal nerve branches. But what is the kinetic and biodynamic occasion? If positional relationships are really important, only those body parts that are capable of being innervated can provide the occasion. It is necessary then to determine the uniqueness of these positional relationships.

At present, there is no information available in man on the molecular relationships between the cell membranes of nerve fibers and the membranes of cells capable of being innervated. Nevertheless, from the developmental kinetic viewpoint one would expect that even the microscopic tip of a growing nerve fiber is a very sensitive structure. It would seem impossible for the tip to be unimportant in the determination of the fiber pathway. What developmental kinetic and (metabolic) biodynamic processes could possibly occur in vivo at the tapered end of a nerve fiber? The embryonic nerve fiber tip is greatly exposed in position and, as it grows it enlarges under unusual conditions. Because of these two factors, the membrane probably is endangered in vivo and is constantly rebuilding and adding to itself. In general, membranes that are not rebuilding are not living and are not found in vivo.

In light of the metabolic ability of the membranes, two molecular movements would be possible in nerve cell processes. The first possibility is that extracellular submicroscopic particles move from outside the cell along or into the cell membranes from which they would move to some extent into the cytoplasm of the nerve cell. A second possibility is the movement of submicroscopic particles in the opposite direction, i.e. from the cytoplasm along the inside of the membranes or into the cell membrane from which they would then move outwards. In both instances, some molecular movements would be parallel to the membrane surface (parmeations) and some would be perpendicular (permeations), thereby causing intracellular fluxion. The authors believe that intracellular fluxion is determined by the developing tips of sensory and motor nerve fibers.

SENSORY FIBER PATHS

When detailed investigations and measurements of anatomical specimens are made from the biokinetic viewpoint, the following concept is reached. First of all, nerve fibers seem to attain different pathways because their origins are different. This appears to be clear-cut and is an important early factor. Because of the different developmental origins of the nerve fibers, their functions are different from the very beginning. The contrasting growth directions of the dorsal and ventral roots described above lead one to conclude that the different functions which nerve fibers later exhibit are predesigned embryologically.

Initially, the anlagen of sensory fiber paths grow only towards thickened ectoderm, e.g. the ectoderm ring (Fig. 7-2). The ultrastructure of the embryonic efferent neurite tip reveals the presence of synapses and presynaptic vesicles both of which indicate permeation-type movements. These ultrastructural features are not present in the tip of embryonic afferent processes. Thus, the position, shape and structure of the tips of sensory conduction pathways differ from those of motor pathways. Usually, only the thickened limiting tissues, e.g. ectoderm ring, ectodermal placodes or ectoderm of face region, are obtained by the tips of growing sensory fibers. An example of this is the medial surface of the limb bud, the thickening of which results from the growth adduction of the limb (Fig. 9-15). Because of the affinity the sensory tips have for thickened ectoderm, there is a good reason to assume that the compressed cells of the thickened ectoderm very likely release metabolic substances into the adjacent intercellular area from where they are absorbed by the membrane at the tip of the sensory fiber (Fig. 9-16, right side). This concept is supported by the

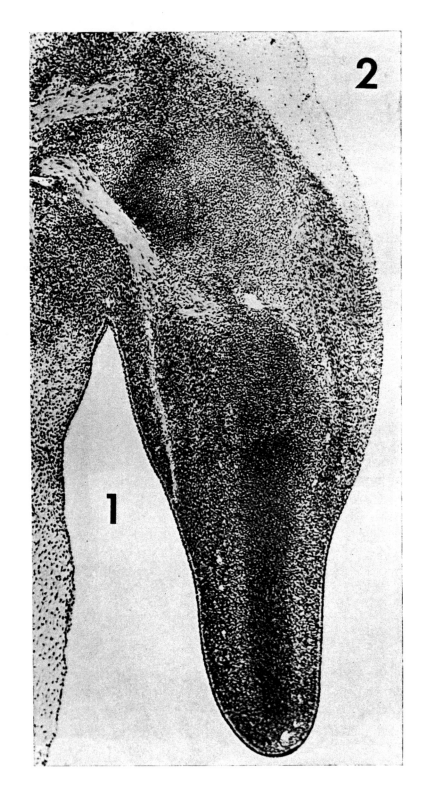

finding that sensory fiber tips (dendrites) extend into small collections of fluid in the innervation zone. In contrast, thin ectoderm has few direct intercellular junctions with the deep inner tissue because of the underlying flattened stroma (Fig. 9-4). The flattening cells and interstices become aligned parallel to the ectodermal surface. The flattened stroma shows no paths to the ectoderm. In accordance with this structure there are initially no paths which provide guiding structures for the nerve fibers.

It is conceivable that at least part of the substances absorbed into the dendrite tip would contribute to the membrane construction at the tip.* In this way, the growing dendrite would be able to lengthen into the innervation zone by the drawing action created by the absorption of such substances (Fig. 9-16, broken line at top right). The molecules that are not used in membrane construction possibly undergo parmeation movement in the cytoplasm along the fiber membrane. This conveyor belt type movement could then move the molecules through the nerve fiber to the vicinity of the ganglioblast nucleus where cell metabolism is centrally controlled. Many details concerning this field are still to be investigated.

From morphology alone one can consider the depressions or concavities on the cell body between the dendrites as zones in the cell membrane where substances are transported toward the cell nucleus (Fig. 9-17). This assumption is supported by the finding that, with the passage of time, afferent synapses become progressively more numerous on the concave portions of the cell membrane. The presynaptic vesicles that are known to occur in these zones are highly suggestive of the movement of substances across the synapse toward the cell nucleus. When the degree of curvature of thin membranes is interpreted as a measure of pressure difference, then the deep depressions of the cell membrane between the dendrites appear as a very important prerequisite for

*This is in accordance with experiments: Bray, D. "Surface Movements during the Growth of Single Explanted Neurons," *Proc. Nat. Acad. Sci. 65*:905-910, 1970.

Figure 9-15. Micrographic section through a 14 mm embryo, stage 18, approximately 6½ weeks, 80× (Blechschmidt Collection), showing the limb bud in longitudinal section. Early sensory innervation is apparent for the thick epithelium (*1*) on the medial side of the limb bud. The thin epithelium (*2*) on the lateral side is without innervation.

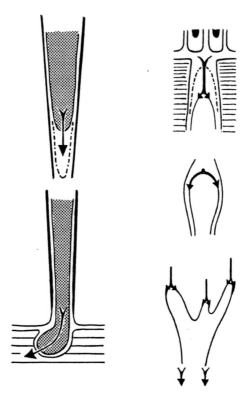

Figure 9-16. Diagrams showing growth movements in the region where motor (left) and sensory (right) nerves arise. Arrows indicate movement of materials on the tips of the growing nerve fibers.

the transmission, of afferent metabolic movements. Such a depression indicates a lower pressure on the inner side of the membrane.

If it is true that functions also undergo development, then this principle should also apply to the development of conduction. This would mean that the membranes of the embryonic nerve fibers already exhibit a primitive conduction of some sort. Perhaps at first, the manner is molecular (submicroscopic) rather than submolecular (electrical). One should not exclude the possible existence of a metabolic gradient between the membranes of the cells that are capable of being innervated and the membranes of the nerve cell processes. The movements of materials in the zones

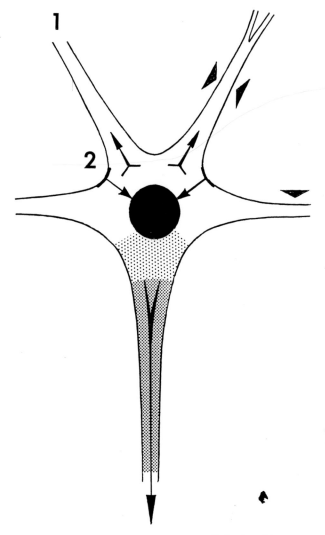

Figure 9-17. Diagram of a human ganglionic cell body with one neurite (ax-on) and several dendrites. In accordance with the growth fluxion in the neu-rites a wrinkling of the cell body becomes established resulting in the for-mation of dendrites. The neurons are parts of a mosaic with star-shaped cells. *1*, region of appositional growth of the dendritic membranes in the manner shown in Figure 9-16 (right); *2*, negative relief of the cell body site where a neighboring cell process reaches the cell body and where movements of particles towards the nucleus are possible. Tailed arrows show direction of metabolic movements (fluxion). Arrowheads indicate pressure differences from outside inwards. Neurite is densely stippled; the cone of the neurite is sparsely stippled.

where conductive pathways arise are surely more delicate than those in the zones where vascular pathways originate. Nevertheless, according to the principle of developmental dynamics, they both have a linearly directed, metabolic gradient in the cycle of metabolism.

MOTOR FIBER PATHS

The following view of the pathfinding process of motor nerve fibers is in accordance with the process discussed for sensory fibers. In any given situation, motor fibers generally grow toward the nearest muscle fiber anlagen, for example myotomes (Fig. 7-4, *3* and Fig. 9-18). Innervation begins at the moment when the muscle fibers are in the process of growth dilation (Chapter 18).

Ultramicroscopic findings have shown that, in later stages of development, substances from the motor neurite tips clearly move toward the periphery. The important finding allows for certain conclusions to be drawn. When muscle fibers lengthen by the process of growth dilation their cell nuclei become arranged into long rows. Fiber lengthening apparently causes the cell nuclei to be displaced as if drawn by suction. Such a suction could conceivably cause local expansion of the outer surface of the growing muscle fiber. This would result in the well-known arrangement of the end plate region where the neurite tip attaches to the muscle fiber. In this instance, molecules would move from the nerve cell body through the neurite and into or through the membranes of the neurite tip (Fig. 9-16, left side). They would thereby bring about appositional growth of the tips and contribute to the development of the muscle fiber. In comparison with embryonic nerves those of an adult appear much thinner and more slender. The growth innervation process is brought about by the relationships between the growing membranes of both the muscle fiber and the neurite. This process is a precursor of the later electrophysiological processes. Growth innervation is very intense and precedes the more complicated physiological innervation process.

If it is assumed that motor innervation is an expression of the metabolic relationships between membranes of both embryonic

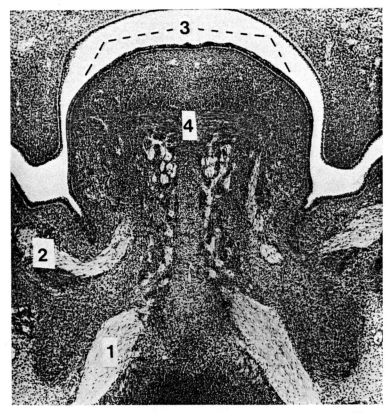

Figure 9-18. Coronal section through a 13 mm embryo, stage 18, approximately 6½ weeks, 60× (Blechschmidt Collection), showing the tongue region in cross section. Development of motor fibers is determined by the position of muscle fiber anlagen. *1*, stem of the hypoglossal nerve branching in the muscle anlagen; *2*, lingual nerve; *3*, thickened epithelium of the tongue; *4*, lingual septum with adjacent tongue muscles.

muscle fibers and nerve cells, then the kinetic processes involved in innervation cannot be exactly the same for the various types of muscle fibers. In light of the kinetic processes described for growth innervation, it is obvious that an extensive innervation would develop in muscle fibers that are lengthening at a rapid pace. Conversely, slowly lengthening fibers, particularly smooth muscle, would receive a less extensive innervation. This is actually what happens.   Observations to the contrary have not been demonstrated.

The apparent kinetic differences between the sensory and motor pathfinding processes can be summarized in the following way. A sensory fiber draws toward substances outside its tip and uses outside molecules to construct its growing membrane whereas a motor fiber transfers intracellular substances into and through its growing tip to the growing muscle fiber and consequently becomes drawn.   This concept is supported by the shape of long nerve cell processes.   It is demonstrated by the observation that the proportions between the surface membrane and the volume of the nerve process change rapidly during development.   The membrane always increases more than the cytoplasm.   This morphology, plus the finding that the nucleus swells in the cell body, strongly suggests that the development of nerve fiber pathways is based on metabolic movements that have a definite spatial order. What is observed in the adult is probably the "remains" of the much more elementary growth functions of the embryo.   There is nothing contradictory in the concept that sensory and motor innervations actually originate as afferent and efferent growth processes, respectively (functional development) (Fig. 9-16) .

MYELINATION

The myelination of nerve fibers cannot be excluded from the uniform process of movements that occur during embryonic development.   Just as it is impossible to disregard the biodynamic functions of the membranes at the fiber tip during the pathfinding process, it follows that consideration should also be given to the biodynamic function of the membranes on the longitudinal surface of the growing fibers.   From all organs that have so far been sufficiently investigated it has been learned that their functional structure is primarily a growth structure which obtains its functional importance only gradually by adaptive processes during growth.   That is why one is motivated to consider also the envelopment of Schwann cells as being a growth architecture.   The longitudinal growth of nerve fibers in situ is consistently characterized by the lengthening of the accompanying Schwann cells.   One wonders why nerve cell processes never rupture in spite of their immense lengthening and corresponding narrowing. What allows embryonic developments of these extreme proportions? It is able to occur because of the assistance of the peripheral glia or Schwann cells.

The investigation of specimens led to the following concept. Serial sections show that Schwann cells grow longitudinally as the nerve fiber lengthens. However, during lengthening, the nodes of Ranvier (constrictions) do not become broader. Lengthening of nerve fibers is not equal throughout. They very likely lengthen in a saltant fashion between the region of Ranvier's nodes. In the area of Ranvier's nodes nutrients can penetrate between the Schwann's sheath and the axon. As the nerve fiber lengthens, the space, and consequently the opportunity, is given to the inner lip of the Schwann cell to envelope the nerve fiber progressively.

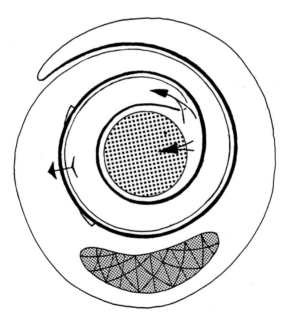

Figure 9-19. Diagram of a myelinated axon (large sparse stipple). The nucleus is densely stippled. Tailed arrows represent metabolic movements.

The occasion for enveloping is due to the low pressure between the borders of the Schwann cell and the lengthening axon (Fig. 9-19, area of the tails of the arrows on the right). The direction of those metabolic movements which pass radially outwards determines the myelination. Figure 9-19 explains that usually the envelopments increase in number as the axon grows and accordingly the rate of isolation of the axons also increases. This interpretation of the observations is in accordance with the finding that only large and firm nerve fibers exhibit intense myelination, but the small nerves do not.

As the number of envelopments increases, the membranes of the Schwann cell enlarge more than its cytoplasm. Older Schwann cells that surround particularly long axons are composed almost entirely of membranes having only a relatively small proportion of cytoplasm.

10

HEAD REGION

No ORGAN HAS BEEN FOUND to be functionless in any phase of its development, including the embryonic anlagen of the organs in the head region. Every body part that can be morphologically delimited as a metabolic field is, at the very least, important in forming activities, i.e. it contributes to the formation of the total organism. Accordingly, every organ system, every organ and every cell aggregation are part of a spatial and kinetic entity. The discussions here are based on this view of the organism. However, such a concept does not exclude other views.

The area between the brain and the cardiac bulge in 2 to 3 mm embryos, i.e. the early lower head region, exhibits typical folds (arches) that cause the lateral part of the body wall to vary considerably in thickness (Fig. 10-1). The folds arise in the lower part of the embryonic head and form a series of arches in accordance with the increased bending of the embryo. The most cranial of the curved folds is the mandibular arch (1) that is the first to form and arises just caudal to the optic vesicle prominence and the adjacent upper jaw anlage. The succeeding folds form in a cranial to caudal sequence giving rise to the second or hyoid arch (2) followed by the third or upper laryngeal arch (3). The fourth or lower laryngeal arch does not appear until near the end of the first month of development.

Since these superficial folds consistently differentiate as part of the bending process of the embryo, they are referred to as "bending folds." Because of their position they also have been called pharyngeal or visceral arches (topographic terms). Investigations into the topokinetics of this area clearly show that the mesenchyma at the base of the mesencephalon becomes transversely aligned (to the longitudinal axis of the embryo) when the embryo bends ventrally. This mesenchyma forms a transverse septum between the forebrain (prosencephalon) and hindbrain (rhombencephalon) (Figs. 10-3 and 10-4). It is called the submesencephalic septum. The notochord lies at the base of the septum and consistently shortens by curving laterally as development proceeds. Occasionally the notochord bifurcates with each segment coursing transversely, following the transversely broadened septum that is established when the embryo bends (Fig. 8-5). The neuromeres (rhombomeres) in the base of the rhombencephalon are also manifestations of the

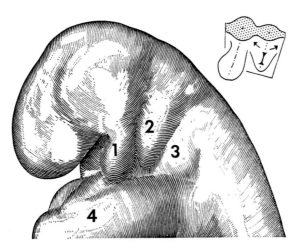

Figure 10-1. Lateral view of the serially reconstructed head region of a 2.57 mm embryo, stage 12, 23 somites, 26 days. The otic vesicle is not yet closed (small light spot). *1,* mandibular or first pharyngeal arch (lower jaw); *2,* hyoid or second pharyngeal arch; *3,* upper laryngeal or third pharyngeal arch; *4,* cardiac prominence. Diagram at upper right shows growth movements of pharyngeal arches. Convergent arrows represent the retarded longitudinal growth resulting from stretched mesenchyma in the interior. Divergent arrows indicate resulting intense circular surface growth.

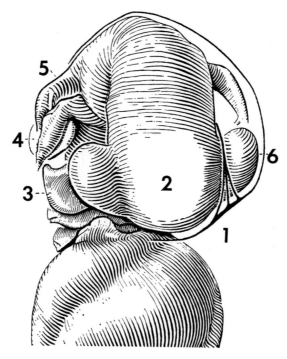

Figure 10-2. Frontal view of the serially reconstructed head region of a 3.4 mm embryo, stage 12, 27 somites, approximately 27 days. *1,* olfactory placode which is caused by stretched mesenchyma that exhibits a restraining function; *2,* forebrain; *3,* endodermal bending fold of the embryo (pharyngeal pouch I); *4,* otic vesicle; *5,* trigeminal nerve; *6,* optic vesicle.

bending process (Fig. 10-4, *2*) . All of these formations are related to each other through their kinetics and particularly through their biodynamics.

In Chapter 8 the paired aortic anlage in the head region was shown to have a restraining function. The longitudinal growth of the anlage does not keep pace with the neural tube but remains short. Because of this, the mesenchymal continuation of the embryonic aorta in the head region becomes stretched (Fig. 8-3). The stretched mesenchyma bridles the brain in this area and causes it to bend, forcing it to arch convexly dorsalward (Fig. 10-3). Thereby, the embryonic face broadens between the brain and the heart

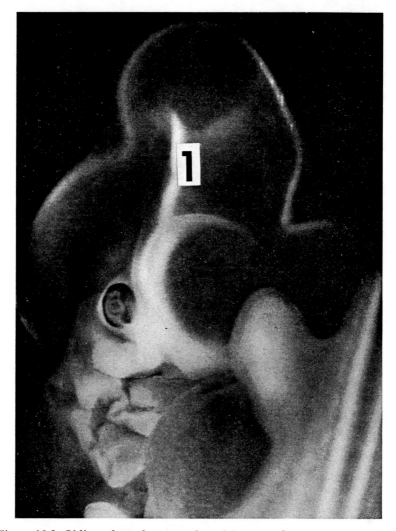

Figure 10-3. Oblique frontal aspect of an 8.8 mm embryo, stage 16, middle of sixth week. 20×. Notice the omega-shape bending of the brain and the submesencephalic septum (*1*).

(Fig. 10-2). The characteristic transverse alignment of the mouth at this stage is consistent with broadening of the face area. As the face broadens, the connective tissue located lateral to the

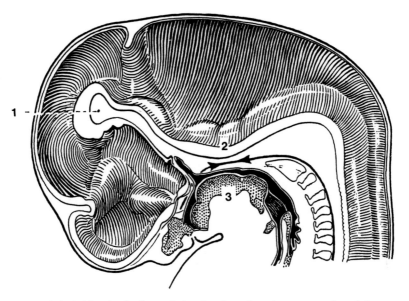

Figure 10-4. Midsagittal view of the head region from a total serial reconstruction of a 10 mm embryo, stage 17, sixth week (Blechschmidt Collection, Carnegie no. 10310). *1*, position of the submesencephalic septum; *2*, neuromeres; *3*, arching endoderm corresponding to the bending brain (anlage of the tongue). Convergent arrows indicate restraining function of the thickened ectomeninx at the base of the brain.

embryonic mouth appears to be stretched in a direction circular to the long axis of the head gut. In 2 mm embryos it is the stroma of the first pharyngeal arch. Cells and intercellular substances in this area align parallel to the direction of the stretch. The stretching causes resistance to the longitudinal (long axis of arch) surface growth of the ectoderm and endoderm in the first pharyngeal arch *(see* Fig. 10-1, convergent arrows in upper right diagram). This phenomenon is manifested by ectoderm and endoderm growth that is circular to the direction of the stretch (Fig. 10-1, divergent arrows in upper right diagram). The unequal surface growth of the first arch causes it to thicken and bulge. As the arch bulges, the first pharyngeal groove[8] and pouch appear on the out-

---

[8]The usual term "cleft" should be avoided, because it implicates the development of an open gill. Real pharyngeal clefts never occur in normal human development.

side and inside of the adjoining walls, respectively. The epithelium lining the groove and pouch is composed of convergent, wedge-shaped cells.

Surface enlargement of the ectoderm and endoderm provides space in the stroma in the interior of the arch for the first aortic arch. It is the first anastomosis between the outflow path of the heart (unpaired ventral aorta) and the paired dorsal aorta (Fig. 8-3). Space for mesenchyma disappears in the area between adjacent pharyngeal arches where the pouch and groove are in contact. The ectoderm in this area is so closely compressed against the endoderm that occasionally a small corrosion field (Chapter 13) develops causing a break or rupture in the wall.

The developmental movements that occur in the upper part of the head region are also determined by the relative position of certain formations. The mesenchyma between the growing optic vesicle and the forebrain bilaterally narrows and becomes stretched (Fig. 10-2). As it stretches its rate of growth becomes less intense. The principle that states that stretched mesenchyma (stroma) acts as a restrainer or restraining apparatus will be explained in Chapter 17. The stretched mesenchyma between the optic vesicle and the forebrain connects to a very small area of ectoderm (anlage of cutis). In this area it functions as a small restraining apparatus. The ectoderm in the restrained area is thereby hindered in surface growth which causes it to thicken, forming the olfactory (nasal) placode or anlage of the nasal pit and nostril (Fig. 10-2, *1*). Comparisons of different regions indicate that limiting tissues such as ectoderm undergo normal thickening when their surface growth is hindered. Among many examples of this are the lens, otic and limb bud placodes. From the developmental kinetic viewpoint, the position of the restraining apparatus for the olfactory placode explains why the nostrils are paired and why they are initially relatively far apart (Fig. 10-5).

In this embryonic period the mesenchymal tissue lateral to the nostrils in the maxillary (infraocular) swelling becomes stretched as the eye expands. This stretched mesenchyma functions as a "hammock" for the eye and courses from the nasal area to the ear

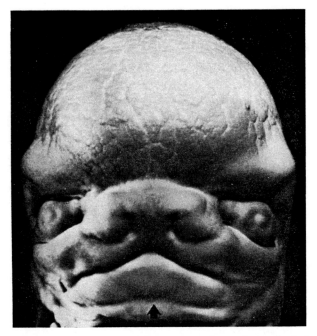

Figure 10-5. Face of a 16.2 mm embryo, stage 19, at the end of the seventh week, 12×. Notice the broad transversely aligned face between the upper head area and the cardiac prominence. Arrowhead indicates growth expansion of the heart. Notice the supranasal sulcus (cf. 1973, p. 86).

as the fibrous zygomatic arch.

Because the metabolic field of the brain determines the development to a great extent, the size of the embryonic cerebral hemispheres is one of the most important prerequisites for total functional development of the organism. At this time, it is necessary to recall the mesenchymal restraining bands (dural girdles) in the cranial ectomeninx that were mentioned in Chapter 9. In the 10 mm embryo the bands are continuous with one another at the base of the brain where the desmal skull is formed (Fig. 10-4, convergent arrows). The early development of these restrainers causes the head to enlarge antibasally, arching convexly, cranialward and forward. Head enlargement is brought about primarily by the formative functions of the brain. Since the ventrally situated endodermal tube (foregut) is a relatively weak structure, it arches convexly cranialward corresponding to the arching pattern of the brain. As a consequence of the arching process, the foregut widens transversely. In addition, an elevation forms on the basal side of the foregut that is more arched than the upper side. This would be expected from the developmental dynamics of the arching process. The elevation is the epithelial anlage of the tongue (Fig. 10-4, *3*). As vaulting of the tongue anlage progresses tridimensionally, musculature develops in its stroma also in all three dimensions, i.e. longitudinal, transverse and vertical (*see* Chapter 18 for the general principle of muscle formation). Since the tongue is a particularly large organ near the brain, a generous cranial nerve innervation would be expected (Fig. 9-18).

The differentiations described above are only a few of numerous ones that accompany formation of the cerebral hemispheres. Cerebralization plays a crucial role in the formation of the upper face area by stretching the related mesenchyma. Such a stretching occurs in the mesenchyma between the eyes causing formation of a transversely aligned supranasal sulcus (Fig. 10-5). This differentiation is important in the developmental kinetics of face formation. It is also necessary for the determination of the direction of sight and for the proportions of the face (Figs. 10-5 and 10-6). The developmental kinetics of face formation will be discussed additionally in Chapter 17. As can be seen from the above figure references, the face of a 16.2 mm embryo appears as a transversely aligned area between the cerebral and cardiac prominences. The space between these two prominences increases as the brain ascends (in relation to the heart) and the heart descends (in relation to the brain). As the intervening space gradually increases in the longitudinal direction, the face area gradually lengthens the same way. It thereby changes from transverse alignment to a longitudinal one (Fig. 10-6). Thus, the characteristic human face is a manifestation of human brain and heart development.

Descent and ascent are also fundamentally important to the development of the complex shape and structure of the alimentary canal in the head region. During eccentric growth of the cerebral hemispheres, the crista galli at the base of the developing skull is

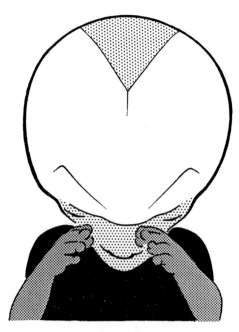

Figure 10-6. Face of a 37 mm fetus, third month. Notice the typical longitudinally aligned face characteristic of the adult.

anchored to the plate-like mesenchyma of the skull by the falx cerebri and the antibasal ectomeninx (dura mater anlage). On the other side, the connective tissue floor of the nasal capsule is connected by way of the stroma in the embryonic cheek region with the cervical portion of the alimentary canal (Fig. 17-5). This portion of the canal is resistant to tension by blood vessels and descends with the hyoid region and the entire laryngotracheal tract. The falx cerebri functions biomechanically as a strong restrainer against the growth pull of the descending viscera. The nasal capsule is caught in the middle of the two opposing forces and is stretched into a muzzle in the vertical plane.

As a result of the increasing distance between the ascending brain and descending viscera, the bilateral tissue in the face region becomes stretched longitudinally and consequently approaches the midline. (it moves in a similar way to a rubber

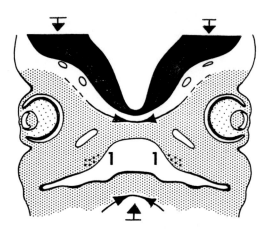

Figure 10-7. Drawing of a coronal section through the head region of a 14 mm embryo, stage 18, approximately 6½ weeks. The face at this time is still broad. Vertical arrows with base lines indicate the main growth expansion of the brain and heart. Converging arrows at the base of the brain represent the restraining function of the basal part of the ectomeninx (dura mater anlage). Converging arrows at the base of the lower jaw region show the restraining function of the pericardium and of the neighboring mesenchyma underneath the cervical sulcus. Large dots represent mesenchymal fibers in the palatine processes (*1*) that are cut transversely and appear stretched in the dorsoventral axis.

ring, circular in diameter, which is stretched to form a narrow gap). During this period the mouth becomes relatively narrow in relation to the total volume of the head. The distances between the angles of the mouth and between the eyes do not keep pace with the increasing size of the head. The distances remain relatively unchanged and narrow. Even though the eyes actually move very little, the floors of the left and right orbits, which form the anlagen of both (lateral) palatine processes approach each

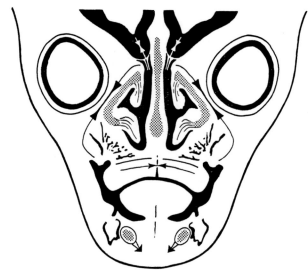

Figure 10-8. Drawing of a coronal section through the head region of a 40 mm fetus, third month. The face lengthens as the brain ascends and the heart and intestines descend. Converging arrows medial to the eyes indicate the restraining function of the mesenchymal nasal capsule. The white arrows represent the restraining function of olfactory nerves. The outlined arrows represent a growth movement (Stemmkörperfunktion) of Meckel's cartilage (contribution to chin formation). The lining epithelium of oral and nasal cavities and the contained fluid are solid black as are the retina and cerebral hemisphere wall. Nasal cartilage is stippled, osseous trabeculae are shown as branching radiants. Converging arrows in the palate area represent the developmental movement of the palatine processes.

other. It is not until the late embryonic period that the dorsoventral dimensions of the face (depth) increase substantially. This growth is manifested by a dorsoventral alignment of the mesenchymal cells lateral to the tongue (dots in Fig. 10-7). From the viewpoint of developmental kinetics, the increase in the depth of the face is constructively related to growth of the cartilaginous lower jaw (Meckel's cartilage) which is directed ventrally (Chapter 16). With dorsoventrally directed facial growth, the stroma of the palatine processes which is the guiding structure of the large blood vessels and nervous pathways of the palate (palatine vessels and nerves) is stretched in its dorsoventral axis (Fig. 10-7, large dots). This stretching results in the anlage of the palatine process that forms below the eye. Initially the process has a convex border with the convexity directed medially and caudally. The palatine process becomes progressively straightened because of the increased dorsoventral stretching. The free border of each process (Fig. 10-7, *1*) undergoes appositional growth because of its divergent wedge epithelium. Continued appositional growth causes the processes to grow medially where they begin to attach to one another in the midline along their free borders. Consequently, the interpalatine space becomes narrower and when closed separates the oral and nasal cavities (Figs. 10-7 and 10-8).

The epithelial lining of the nasal capsule initially has an oval shape. As the surrounding tissue is stretched dorsoventrally, the lining epithelium (mucosa) becomes so compressed that it bends into folds forming the nasal conchae anlagen (Fig. 10-8). The conchae anlagen enlarge differently in accordance with their position. It is only after the shape of the desmal conchae is established and they enlarge considerably that their cartilaginous and osseous skeleton appears in the interior. It is contrary to the facts to think that the skeleton is formed first, and then the mucosa of the conchae appears as a "protector" of the skeleton.

Because of changes in the proportion of the whole face, space becomes available which is prerequisite for all of the described differentiations that occur there. Changes in the face proportions are brought about by the ascent and descent of the larger organ systems of the embryo. In this sense, the human face is an expression of the development of brain and heart.

11

TRUNK

In this chapter the relationship between the development of the trunk wall and the development of the viscera will be particularly emphasized. Investigations repeatedly show that descent of the viscera is a movement which is very basic to intestinal tract development. This descent contributes to the developmental movements of the entire embryo in a very important way. Caudal movement of the viscera is referred to as descent primarily relative to the brain. A well-known manifestation of visceral descent is the innervation of the diaphragm by the phrenic nerve that arises from spinal cord segment C4. In another aspect of developmental movement the entire neural tube could be viewed as ascending (cranial movement of the neural tube relative to the intestinal tube). A typical example of ascent is the progressive formation of the cauda equina from the roots of the lumbar and sacral spinal nerves which course vertically in the vertebral canal. Another example is the progressive protrusion of the embryonic forehead at the upper end of the neural tube.

The question of what causes viscera to descend during development is a very interesting one. One of the most remarkable biodynamic factors that apparently initiates this movement is growth of the embryonic liver on the underside of the diaphragm anlage. The earlier development of the heart and brain seem to be very important prerequisites for liver growth. Intense growth of the brain is necessarily accompanied by intense vascularization. As vascularization increases the early heart must enlarge which causes it to become the central mass of the vascular system. As the heart progressively enlarges blood flow to it progressively increases. This causes the liver to enlarge since it is the most proximal area to the heart. Venous blood collects here and is the first supplier of blood to the enlarging heart which is the center of the vascular system. The liver appears to function as a filter for blood before it courses to the heart. The liver thereby develops into the central mass of the intestinal tract. As the heart and liver gradually enlarge the stroma between them becomes compressed into a plate of tissue. This is caused by the expansion growth of both organs. Actually, the tissue of the diaphragm appears as a severely compressed thin layer between the heart and the liver. At the beginning of the second month the compression seems so intense that the intermediate layer progressively thins, contains little blood and has a pale appearance (cf. 1975, figures on pp. 83, 143, 217, 281). Thus the layer differentiates into the anlage of the central tendon of the diaphragm. Only the more peripheral part of the diaphragm differentiates into long muscle fiber bundles as the circumference of the trunk increases. These bundles form the muscular margin (margo muscularis) of the diaphragm.

Even in the 4.2 mm embryo the importance of liver growth in causing the diaphragm anlage to dome is already evident. The liver anlage at this time is located high in the cervical region dorsal to the heart (Fig. 11-1, right drawing). Initially, it is small but already clearly arched in a convex manner cranialward. Later, in the 10 mm embryo it has enlarged considerably and lies caudal to the heart (Fig. 11-1, left drawing). By the seventh week (17.5 mm), the liver moves more and more ventralward where it contributes to the increasing circumference of the trunk. This is especially noticeable in the region of the lower thoracic aperture (Fig. 11-2). Here again there is a characteristic topokinetics (position kinetics) that is closely related to both a specific morpho-

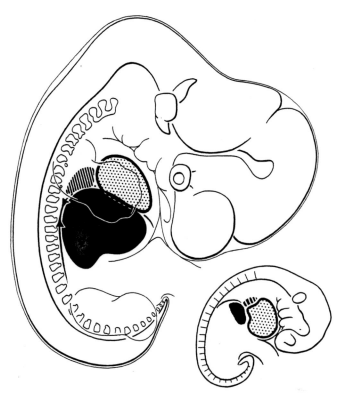

Figure 11-1. Scale drawings taken from serial reconstructions of 4.2 mm (right) and 10 mm (left) embryos showing the development of the lungs in the paravertebral heart-liver angle. Liver is black, heart is stippled and pleura is striped. Convergent arrows in the 10 mm embryo show the restraining function of the diaphragm.

kinetics (shape kinetics) and tectokinetics (structure kinetics).

As the liver expands, the dome of the diaphragm anlage flattens by moving caudally and ventrally, i.e. toward the umbilical area (cf. 1975, pp. 51, 115, 167, 249). In this way the diaphragm anlage gives up its original position behind the heart and detaches caudally from its position in front of the cervical portion of the embryonic vertebral column. It descends progressively also from the thoracic portion of the vertebral column and the adjoining ribs. During the movement the diaphragmatic tissue gradually

remains in contact with the developing skeleton only in the region
of the lumbar vertebral column and the lower thoracic aperture
(Fig. 11-2). Comparison of Figures 11-1 and 11-2 shows that as this
developmental movement occurs the angle increases between the

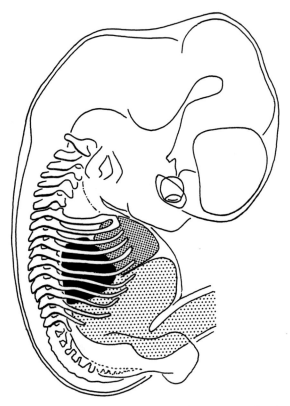

Figure 11-2. A 17.5 mm embryo showing the developmental relations of the
thoracic wall to the heart-liver mass and to the lung. Broken line in the
neck region represents the sternocleidomastoid muscle (see 1973 for additional illustrations).

paravertebral portions of the heart and liver (heart-liver angle)
thereby providing space for the expanding pleural sacs and lungs
(cf. 1973, pp. 53, 107).

In the region of the mediastinum the pericardium and heart
move caudally with the diaphragm. All of the cervical viscera in

turn move caudally with the heart. Externally, the descent of cervical viscera is evident by the configuration of the embryonic neck region (Fig. 11-3). Descent of the large heart from the cervical region into the thorax brings about substantial spatial changes in the neck region. These spatial changes are so great that the wall of the neck region collapses relative to the cranial and thoracoabdominal walls. The narrowness of the adult neck should remind us of the fundamental movements during the embryonic period, i.e. descent of viscera and ascent of the central nervous system. The trunk of the embryo becomes erect as the cartilaginous vertebral column becomes stronger and firmer. The more the embryo becomes erect, the more distinct the embryonic neck appears. The general features of differentiating cartilage are given in Chapters 15 and 16.

There are still other features related to the above developmental movements. Many of them will be pointed out in subsequent chapters. It is sufficient to say here that all of the differ-

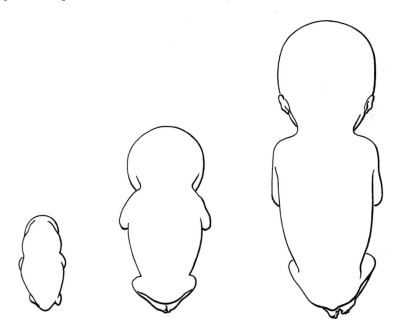

Figure 11-3. Back views of 16 mm, 30 mm and 43 mm specimens showing the formation of the neck as the intestines descend and the trunk erects.

entiation processes in the trunk region are in complete biodynamic harmony with each other. Differentiations should not be viewed phylogenetically merely as recapitulations—this does not explain how they form. Neither should one view differentiations genetically as coming from patterns that are preformed in the genes. A thorough understanding of differentiations can only be obtained through developmental dynamics.

In Chapter 8 it was noted that without knowing the developmental dynamics of descent and ascent it would not be possible to describe the origin of the thyroid gland and the hypophysis as interrelated processes. The origin of these ductless glands would forever remain a mystery without a knowledge of the surrounding processes which determine them. Close and thorough examination of developmental movements consistently confirms the principle that the development of the internal (cell) structure of an organ cannot be divorced from the development of its outer shape which, in turn, is inseparable from the development of its position. Descent and ascent are developmental movements which clearly show that position, shape and structure are but momentary aspects of performances in varying orders of magnitude. These three aspects of performances have a much closer correlation than do processes that are causally related.

It was shown in Chapter 10 that the ascent and descent of the large organ systems of the embryo are prerequisites for the differentiations in the head region. This is also true for the trunk viscera, especially the lungs. In contrast to the nasal portion of the respiratory tract, the bronchopulmonary portion develops under another set of circumstances. Development of the respiratory tract in the paravertebral heart-liver angle during enlargement of the thorax is an early complex movement. This movement could be viewed as the first "breathing" movement. Many investigators seem to have the erroneous idea that organ systems are formed first and then, after their formation, their useful functions are affixed seemingly by addition. The so-called first breath of the newborn infant is but a stage in the long development of breathing actions that begin with the origin of the lungs. *Functions can be exerted postnatally only when they have begun as growth functions in the prenatal period.* This is the principle by which these conclusions have been reached.

Growth of the brain with its many closely packed cells causes the blood circulation to enlarge additionally. Enlargement of the circulation field causes the heart to increase in size. If the brain would not have enlarged early (cerebralization of the embryo), there would not be the occasion for increased growth of the heart (cardialization of the embryo). If growth of the heart did not increase, blood flow to the heart would not increase. Consequently, the liver would not expand (hepatization). Increased hepatic growth causes the circumference of the liver to increase. The increase in the liver circumference in turn causes the diaphragm to flatten which is very important for descent of the viscera and the resulting origin of the nasal and bronchopulmonary portions of the respiratory tract. As is evident from this, developmental processes occur step by step. *The origin of organs is consistently the beginning of the development of their functions.*

At this time a short remark should be made about the development of the ribs and the differentiation of the ventral thoracic wall. Preformed guiding structures must accompany the longitudinal growth of the ribs. The mesenchyma within the embryonic trunk wall is strongly stretched circularly only at the periphery of the heart-liver bulge. Only in this zone does the stretched mesenchyma appear to be the guiding structure for the growing ribs (Chapter 14). Stretching of the mesenchyma varies locally in accordance with the unequal quick expansion of the heart-liver bulge. This explains how individual ribs develop differing lengths and why ribs are normally absent in the cervical and lumbar regions.

The tendon of the stenocleidomastoid muscle passes bilaterally into the ventral thoracic wall (Fig. 11-2). The growth pull of the tendons causes the ventral segment of the ventrally growing ribs to converge. On each side they fuse with the respective sternocleidomastoid tendon. Paired sternal bars are formed in this way corresponding to the paired muscle. The primarily desmal sternal bars subsequently fuse in the midline to form the sternum. Where the circumference of the liver is greatest, fusion of the sternal bars is retarded. The ribs in this region diverge more and more ventralward and caudalward. The caudal ribs terminate freely in the surrounding, less stretched connective tissue (Fig. 11-2). In summary, it is apparent that even in the embryonic stages the thoracic wall and lungs are functionally closely related to the heart and liver.

If it is truly a principle that the origin of organs is also the beginning of their function, then it must be possible to apply this principle to other growth functional systems. If it is true for central organs like the heart and liver, it should also be true for retroperitoneal organs. The development of the kidney will be described as another example of this principle. Is the origin of the kidney also the beginning of its characteristic function? The results of these investigations also support the concept that development of the position, shape and structure of organs cannot be separated from the development of their functions. Regularly prenatal growth functions are necessary prerequisites for postnatal functions.

After close observation, it becomes apparent that even the first microscopic anlage of the kidney has the natural plan of the adult kidney with regard to its position, shape and structure, In 9 to 10 mm embryos the kidney is already a retroperitoneal, "kidney-" or bean-shaped organ with upper and lower poles and three layers, i.e. capsule, cortex and medulla (Figs. 11-4 and 11-5) (cf. 1975, pp. 157, 159).

In accordance with the earlier statement that differentiations begin on the outside rather than on the inside and, thus, are always outer modifications of the anlagen, one must first determine what the outer circumstances are in the region where the kidney arises. In addition, and in order to be consistent with previous statements, one would again expect the origin of the kidney to be an embryonic function that is brought about by position. This will be shown to be the case.

During the period when the neural tube lengthens, growth of the great vessels becomes retarded. This includes retarded growth of the paired veins in the trunk wall, i.e. postcardinal veins (Fig. 11-4). Consequently, the distance between the growing neural tube and its adjoining vascular bundles increases. The principle in effect here was examined previously in Chapter 8. Because the paired trunk wall veins remain short, they detach and move ventrally away from the neural tube. The mesonephric (Wolffian) duct, which is attached by tissue to the trunk wall veins, follows

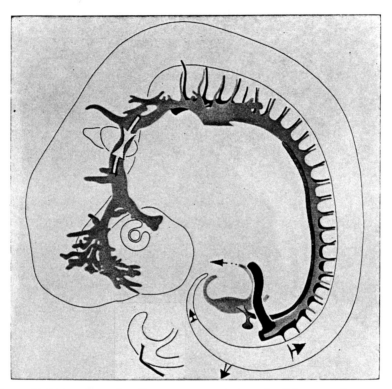

Figure 11-4. Drawing taken from a reconstruction of a 6.3 mm embryo, stage 14, 30 days, (Blechschmidt Collection, Carnegie no. 10308) showing the kinetics pertinent to the initiation of kidney development. Converging white arrows represent the restraining function of the cardinal veins. Arrows with base lines show growth direction of neural tube. Outlined arrow indicates direction of neural tube movement as it unfolds. Arrow at the end of allantois indicates the growth pull of the blood vessels in the umbilical cord. The anlage of the kidney (metanephrogenic diverticulum) arises in a growth zone where there is apparent reduced tissue pressure by enlargement of the space between the neural tube and urogenital sinus. The diagram shows detail of the reconstruction of the 4.2 mm embryo. The bent Wolffian duct is black.

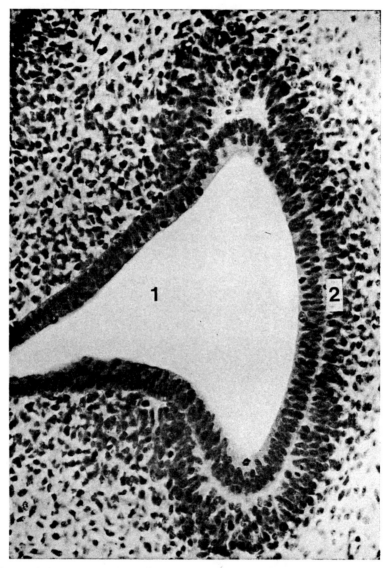

Figure 11-5. A sagittal section through the kidney anlage of a 9.5 mm embryo, stage 17, six weeks, 300×. *1*, transition between embryonic renal pelvis and anlage of renal calices; *2*, metanephrogenic mass (cortex) (cf. 1961, 1973 for additional figures).

the movement of the veins. Near the caudal end of the embryo the duct becomes more and more aligned as a cord of the long, curved neural tube (the arrows in Fig. 11-4 show the developmental movements). Due to these movements the cranial portion of the mesonephric duct is bent against its caudal portion near the urinary bladder anlage (Fig. 11-4).

Serial reconstructions of the total embryo in which the mesonephric duct is demonstrated show that as the caudal segment of the curved neural tube rolls out (Fig. 11-4, lowest arrow), space becomes available between neural tube and urogenital sinus into which the prism-shaped cells of the mesonephric duct grow. The cells grow in the direction of least resistance thereby forming the metanephrogenic diverticulum. The diverticulum arises where the duct is most acutely bent. The surface of the diverticulum then enlarges in the direction of least resistance, i.e. longitudinally and parallel to growth of the entire embryo.

There are several indications that the early embryonic kidney is already functioning as an early excretory organ. Like every normal limiting tissue, the epithelial anlage of the metanephros has two surfaces. One surface is adjacent to fluid and the other is attached to more solid tissue. However, in this instance a unique situation exists. The fluid contained in the kidney-shaped diverticulum is in communication through the lumen of the mesonephric duct with the fluid in the lumen of the embryonic urinary bladder. From there, it is possible for the fluid to diffuse into the blood vessels of the umbilical cord. In other words, permeability of the embryonic renal epithelium is particularly important for the development of its excretory function. Such permeability, together with the formation of the diverticulum, would give this epithelium and its stroma the ability to quickly release katabolites into the lumen of the diverticulum (Fig. 11-6, tailed arrow). As this process takes place, the tissue becomes unburdened and enabled to intensify its metabolism. Morphological studies (counting of mitoses and cells) make it evident that the surface of the entire epithelial renal anlage undergoes intense growth as a result of increased cell proliferation and cell enlargement.

In the second month the vascular supply of the kidney is al-

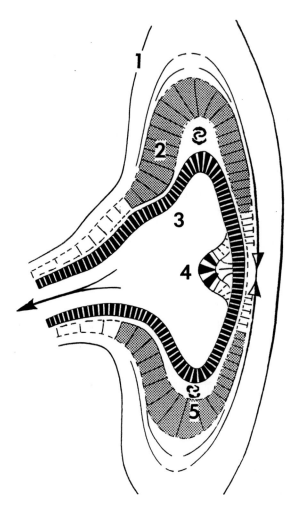

Figure 11-6. Diagram of the developing kidney anlage showing the main directions of the cell limiting membranes. *1*, capsule; *2*, cortex area; *3*, medulla area. Large-tailed arrow shows flow of fluid wastes toward the urogenital sinus (urinary bladder anlage). Convergent arrows peripheral to the cortex area represent the local growth resistance (restraining function) of the renal capsule. To the right of *4* is the infolding epithelium that initiates the formation of the embryonic ureteric tree (ureteric spur).   Above *5* is a mitotic figure.

ready laid down between the cortex and the medulla. As was shown above, the formation of blood vessels is consistently guided in the zone of origin by material movements that are spatially ordered. These findings are therefore good reasons for the assumption that, during the development of functions, nutritive substances are conducted from the renal hilus area not by permeation but by parmeation along the basement membrane of the renal epithelium. The nutritive substances would then be assimilated at the basement membrane. These metabolic movements begin even when there are not yet blood vessels. They are determined by the metabolic gradient. Possibly the adjacent inner tissue also assimilates nutritive substances along the basement membrane. Not only do the number of cells in this area increase but also their volume. As a result, the stroma becomes crowded with cells forming the metanephrogenic mass or cap adjacent to the epithelial renal anlage (Figs. 11-5 and 11-6). The metanephrogenic mass constitutes the cortex of the renal anlage. The cells of the limiting tissue (epithelium) and those of the adjacent inner tissue (mesenchyma) are multiplying and growing causing them to become closely pressed against each other in their respective layers. As a result, the cells in each layer align perpendicular to the basement membrane. The alignment of the cells to the basement membrane can be viewed as a trajectory structure with spatially ordered metabolic movements in the cycle of the metabolism. There are no indications here of diffuse metabolic movements. Without spatially ordered metabolic movements the vascularization would not be conceivable. The katabolites permeate perpendicularly the cell limiting membranes and pass from the cytoplasm of the cells into the lumen of the enlarging kidney diverticulum, i.e. in the direction of least resistance.

Because of their perpendicular alignment to the basement membrane (Fig 11-6), the cells necessarily diverge toward the adjacent stroma where the epithelium bends. This occurs more at the poles of the diverticulum (cranial and caudal ends) than it does between the poles. In this manner, the epithelium becomes wedge-shaped with cell limiting membranes which exhibit a divergence that varies from one location to another. Because the cell limits show different degrees of divergence (differing degrees of wedge epithelium), longitudinal growth of the epithelium occurs at locally different rates. It is intense at the poles but slow between the poles where the wall of the hollow anlage is thin and weak (Fig. 11-6). The circumference of the metanephros enlarges rapidly near the poles whereas the longitudinal sides of the renal anlage flatten.

The epithelial renal medulla is established first, followed by the cortex. Lastly, the capsule differentiates peripheral to the cortex. The limiting membranes of the capsule cells become progressively more tangentially aligned to the cells of the embryonic cortex (Fig. 11-7). Again, the cell membranes exhibit a main direction. The capsule differentiates peripherally in accordance with the surface growth of the medulla together with that of the cortex. As the surface area of the renal anlage increases, the capsule tissue is stressed.

A study of the structural arrangements of the renal anlage again indicates that the formative and developmental functions of its solid and fluid components are very important. Surface growth of the epithelial renal anlage results in the increased production of fluid waste products (embryonic preurine). It is known that such fluid wastes do not usually stagnate in vivo but show movement. To be consistent with this fact, it must be that fluid wastes move to the embryonic urinary bladder where they then diffuse through the wall of the bladder into the umbilical vessels. With this concept, such liquid would be constantly produced and absorbed.

When fluid wastes move toward the urinary bladder, the longitudinal wall of the renal anlage is particularly stressed. This could be compared to the stress placed on a dome by increasing its surface area. The top of such a dome would gradually break down, as does the renal wall forming a spur-like projection (Fig. 11-6). There are few mitoses in the region of the projection. This finding suggests that the renal wall in this area is passively compressed from the sides. This would not only cause the projection to lengthen but would also cause increased necrosis within it. Establishment of the spur-like projection initiates the forma-

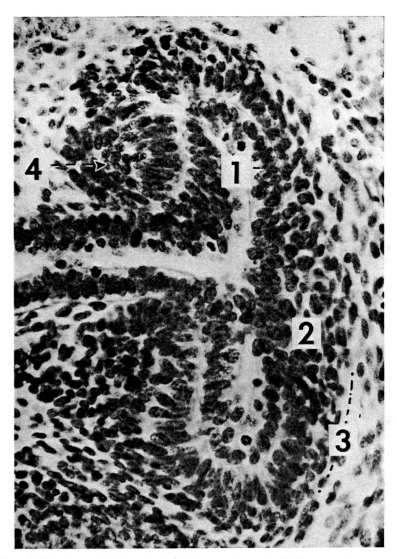

Figure 11-7. A section through the kidney anlage of a 20.5 mm embryo, stage 20, eight weeks. 450×. Three layers, medulla area *(1)*, cortex area *(2)* and capsule area *(3)* are distinct. Spherical cells in area *4* are the region of glomerulus formation.

tion of the ureteric tree subdividing the renal anlage. Necroses would assist in the widening of the renal lumen where calices give rise to collecting ducts.

The kinetic principles for differentiation of the nephrons are relatively simple and are illustrated in Figures 11-7 to 11-9. These figures show that subdivision of the renal anlage leads to formation of anchor-shaped structures that have a lumen. The limiting membranes of the mesenchymal cells on the concave side of the "anchor arms" align primarily in a radial direction to the center of a group of other mesenchymal cells (Figs. 11-7 and 11-8). The central cells have no orientation pattern but become spherical and form mitoses. When their proliferative activity is over, they enlarge and push apart from one another. Lumen formation becomes apparent. Fluid collects in the lumen. The

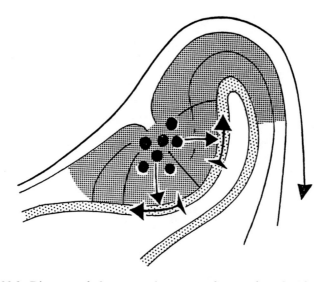

Figure 11-8. Diagram of the zone where a nephron arises showing the trajectorial alignment of the limiting membranes of cells radially arranged around a central collection of spherical cells (large black dots). Diverging arrows with base line show expansion growth of the epithelium of the ureteric tree anlage. Arrows radiating from the collection of spherical cells represent the growth pull of cell limiting membranes due to which the inner cells are under less pressure. Peripheral arrow indicates growth pull direction of the capsule.

cells bordering the accumulated fluid become a limiting tissue. It is in this manner that the embryonic nephrons become apparent. The end segment of the embryonic nephron located between the ureteric tree and the renal capsule thickens and becomes blunt (Fig. 11-9). This segment is the epithelial anlage of the glomerulus. Its outer surface that is adjacent to the ureteric tree becomes extended in surface area together with the growing renal epitheli-

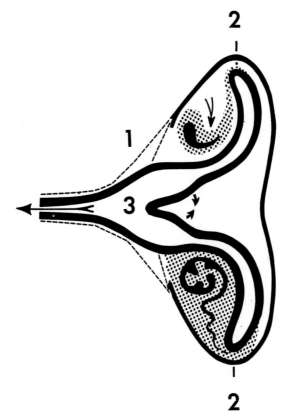

Figure 11-9. Diagram of the kidney anlage showing the relations of the ureteric tree anlage and the nephrons. Broken lines indicate the yielding portions of the capsule area (*1*). Tailed arrows show the direction of material movements. Converging curved arrows represent the direction of movement of the epithelium when forming a spur of the ureteric tree; *2*, site of the corrosion field that subsequently appears between the nephron and the ureteric tree; *3*, transition between the embryonic renal pelvis and calices.

um. It enlarges apparently because of its close relationship to the growing renal epithelium (divergent arrows in Fig. 11-8). Bowman's capsule arises from this area. That portion of the glomerulus anlage that is hindered in surface growth and consequently not thinned folds on itself thereby forming lobulated areas. The stroma of each lobule gives rise to a vascular loop which later becomes a vascular tuft of the glomerulus.

The other end segment of the embryonic nephron narrows sharply and makes very close contact with the epithelium of the ureteric tree (Fig. 11-9, 2). That part of the nephron anlage between its blunt and narrow ends forms the system of tubules. Once a lumen appears throughout the nephron, its walls become a limiting tissue. The prism-shaped, wedge epithelium composing the walls enables the nephron to grow rapidly with a preference in the longitudinal direction of the tubule anlage (*see* Chapter 5). As the tubule lengthens, the basement membrane lengthens also mainly in the longitudinal direction. Simultaneous with this, the basement membrane appears to shorten and strengthen in the transverse plane of the tubule. This would cause the tubules to resist deformation. When the narrow end of the nephron anlage lengthens, it makes contact with one of the branches of the ureteric tree. Such contact sets up a corrosion field (Chapter 13) where two epithelial layers are compressed together resulting in necrosis. In this manner the lumen of the nephron becomes continuous with the lumen of the ureteric tree.

The kinetic principles in effect during kidney development can be summarized as follows. The cells of the renal (metanephrogenic) diverticulum are not aligned tangential but rather perpendicular to the basement membrane. This strongly suggests that the developing wall of the diverticulum is not expanded by the fluid pressure in the lumen of the diverticulum (which appears distended in vivo) but by active surface growth of the cells composing the wall of the diverticulum. Consideration of the developmental dynamics leads to the supposition that a relatively low pressure exists in the growing hollow renal anlage in vivo. This would cause fluid to be released from the wall into the lumen of the ureter-kidney anlage. Thus, the initial formation of the kidney already shows a metabolic gradient that is spatially ordered which in turn gives rise to spatially directed metabolic movements. From this it is apparent that kidney development conforms to the principle that *the origin of organs is also the beginning of their function.* This is an important statement.

Kidney differentiation is a performance that is brought about by the developmental dynamics of the total embryo. The later excretory function of the kidney would be inconceivable without this preliminary function. It is unnecessary to determine whether kidney developmental activity is a recapitulation of the processes of phylogenetic development. The kidney of the human embryo is a uniquely human organ in each period of its development.

12

LIMBS

POSITION AND SHAPE OF THE EARLY LIMB

THE FOUR EXTREMITIES originate in the first month of development as microscopically visible anlagen that have a precise location (Figs. 12-1 and 12-2). They first make their appearance lateral to the angular area between the neural tube and the mesothelial lining of the coelom. Not only do the right and left but also the upper and lower buds differ from one another from the very beginning by this position. As a result of their position they are a part of both the ventral and dorsal walls. Because of this alone one should expect the developmental dynamics of the ventral and dorsal walls to play a very important role in the origin of the extremities. On the other hand, the extremities seem to mediate the different developmental movements of the two walls which are contrasting ways of development. Movement of the ventral wall gives rise to the axillary and inguinal fossae while movement of the dorsal wall gives rise to the appendage elevations.

Both the upper and the lower angles between the neural tube and the coelomic lining have distinct characteristics. The upper one opens cranialward while the lower one opens caudalward (Figs. 12-1 and 12-2). The large postcardinal vein in the wall lies along the medial aspect of the dorsal border of the coelom (cf. 1975, pp. 80-87 and 94-97). During formation of the angles this

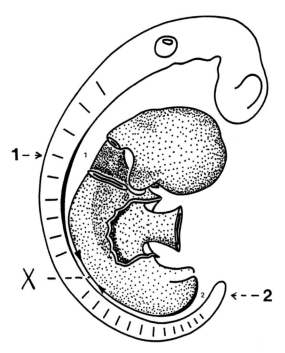

Figure 12-1. Serial reconstruction of a 2.57 mm embryo, stage 12, 23 somites, approximately 26 days showing relationships of serosa (stipple) to neural tube. Limb anlagen appear at level of upper (*1*) and lower (*2*) angles between neural tube and coelomic cavity lining. Converging arrows near "x" represent relative shortening of the dorsal border of the peritoneum along the postcardinal veins.

vein and the coelomic lining both move away from the neural tube cranially and caudally (Fig. 12-2, areas of heavy black lines dorsal to coelom). As this movement takes place, the dorsal metameric branches of the postcardinal vein which are joined to the ectomeninx must lengthen in the region of the angles (Fig. 12-3). When the intersegmental branches lengthen and the neural tube bends, the branches diverge more and more toward the neural tube. Conversely, the branches converge away from the neural tube toward the coelom. Growth of the body wall surface appears retarded in the area where convergence is greatest. This occurs in the surface just superficial to the concave side of the postcardinal

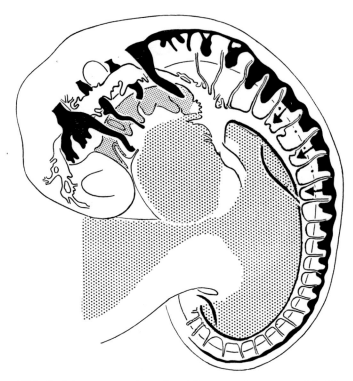

Figure 12-2. Serial reconstruction of a 4.2 mm embryo, stage 13, 30 somites, approximately 28 days showing positional relationships of limb anlagen to the peritoneum and neural tube. Arrows indicate the effect of the convergent growth pull of the metameric veins.

vein. The vein necessarily remains shorter than the neural tube to which it is connected. Because of this vein-neural tube connection, the vein exerts a restraining function against the neural tube. As one would expect, the overlying ectoderm that is hindered in surface growth thickens to form the so-called limb placode (Fig. 12-3, finely stippled area). Other examples of such thickening of hindered epithelium have been given and are consistently evident.

How is the limb bud elevation produced? The ectoderm along the dorsal edge of the placode (Fig. 12-3, largely stippled area) seems to be elevated by the adjacent stroma which is pushed convergently ventralwards (convergent zones in Fig. 12-3) because of

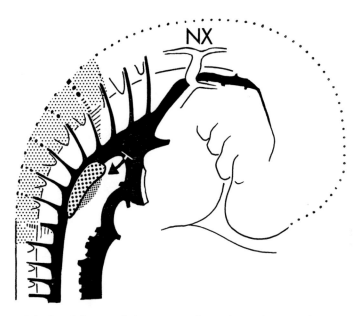

Figure 12-3. Cranial part of the same embryo shown in Figure 12-2 showing the establishing of limb anlage. Loosely stippled area indicates position of the positive relief (projection) of the upper limb anlage. Smaller, densely stippled ventral area shows position of the negative relief (depression) of the anlage where the limb placode is located. Arrow indicates hindered surface growth of the limb placode.

the eccentric growth of the spinal cord and is also helped by the veins which are retarded in growth. In this zone the dermatomes clearly converge toward the postcardinal vein (stippled dorsal area in Fig. 12-3) similar to the way in which the dorsal metameric veins converge toward the limb placode. Both occur at the level of the neural tube-serosa angle near the mesothelium. The early cutis in this narrow area is compressed and appears to move outward along the dorsal edge of the placode thereby forming an elevation (Fig. 12-4). As the elevation arises the placode along with its underlying tissue is pushed medially, thereby forming a depression. The depression is so deep that the body wall protrudes inwardly (Fig. 12-4, arrow with outlined stem). In the upper limb bud the depression represents the early embryonic

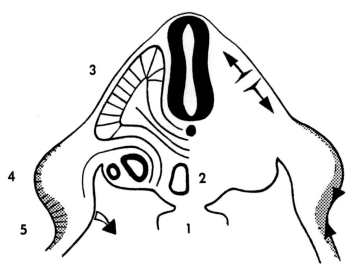

Figure 12-4. Drawing of a transverse section through the upper limb fold region of a 3.7 mm embryo, stage 12, approximately 27 days. *1,* mesentery; *2,* still paired aorta; *3,* lateral trunk wall with dermatome; *4,* positive relief of limb anlage; *5,* negative relief of limb anlage. Divergent arrows show location of accelerated growth of dermatomes and overlying ectoderm. Convergent arrows indicate location of hindered surface growth of ectoderm (placode region). Arrow with outlined stem represents inward protrusion of trunk wall.

axilla. In the lower limb bud it is the early embryonic inguinal region. The elevations are the anlagen of the limbs proper. Before the end of the first month the limb buds become longitudinal folds with flexion and extension sides.

The upper limb bud in 4 to 5 mm embryos can be viewed as a folding that is modified in accordance with its position. The fold in these specimens begins to cover the axillary depression. This movement is brought about because the base of the fold is relatively compact dorsally where there is no coelom, but weak ventrally where it lies adjacent to coelomic fluid (cf. 1975, p. 85). When growth of the surface ectoderm increases, the ventral side of the fold sinks. As a result, the entire fold tilts ventrally thereby covering over the axillary depression. All of the limb buds exhibit a sort of growth adduction with this tilting movement (Figs. 12-5

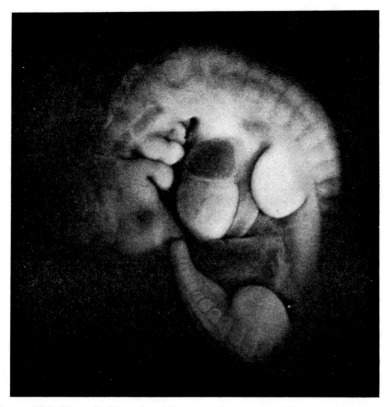

Figure 12-5. Lateral view of a 4.5 mm embryo, stage 13, approximately 29 days, showing upper and lower limb anlagen. There are distinct differences between the two anlagen with elbow and knee areas characterized by clearly different margins.

and 12-6). The upper limb buds are adducted toward the liver bulge; the lower limb buds are adducted toward the root of the umbilical cord.

As the limb anlage adducts, it flattens in the following manner. During the described tilting, the base of the limb bud remains nearly constant in the transitional region where the bud joins the body wall. Thereby the ectoderm on both the extension and flexion sides of the fold become more closely approximated towards each other as tilting occurs. In this manner, the distal part

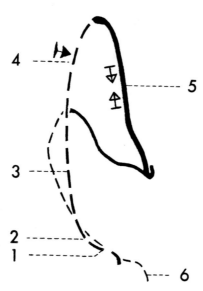

Figure 12-6. Outline of the longitudinal aspect of the upper limb anlage in 7.5 mm and 8 mm embryos showing its positional change. Growth adduction is clearly evident (solid black arrow). Convergent arrows represent hindered growth of the ectoderm on the flexion side of the anlage. *1,* shoulder area; *2,* elbow area; *3,* forearm area; *4,* hand area; *5,* thickened ectoderm; *6,* thin ectoderm.

of the limb fold becomes characteristically paddle-shaped.   During the transformation the extension side lengthens relative to the flexion side or, in other words, the flexion side shortens relative to the extension side.   As a result of this developmental movement, the ectoderm and adjacent stroma become thinner on the extension side and thicker on the flexion side.   This movement is another example of the close relationship that exists between position, shape and structure during development.   Such movements are much more precise than one would expect at first glance.

The tilting of the limb fold with the resulting covering over of the placode is characterized by different speeds of movement in all three dimensions, i.e. craniocaudally, proximodistally and mediolaterally.   The proximal and distal portions of the limb buds develop differently.   Between these two portions a typical connecting piece appears. In the upper limb anlage the proximal portion forms the embryonic shoulder. The distal portion narrows to form the elbow area. The arm segment of the upper extremity is thereby established between these two areas. In other words, in the early stages the entire upper limb anlage really is only the arm segment of the upper extremity. The shoulder and elbow areas of the upper limb anlage become distinct first. This is also true of the embryonic hip and knee areas of the lower limb anlage. Initially, these regions were undefined parts of the early cutis on the lateral trunk wall. Such developmental relations lead to the conclusion that the cutis is the prime mover in the shaping of the limb anlagen.

The intense surface growth of the ectoderm during early development appears to have an important forming function. During development the surface of the limb becomes relatively larger in comparison with the volume of the stromal core. That is why the limb anlage may be considered for a moment as being similar to a tube under low pressure. Due to low pressure the tube is compressed from the outside (Fig. 12-6, black arrow). The growing ectoderm would thereby have the effect of a mold which biodynamically draws its mesenchymal contents from the trunk wall. This performance appears to be an important event in the first period of limb formation when the limb anlage is short (proximodistally) and just begins to flatten. It would thereby prepare the limb anlage for the ingrowth of nerve pathways and blood vessels into the shoulder and hip regions. This idea is consistent with the concept that nerves and blood vessels are pulled structures. Neither structure has the ability to develop normally by itself. They must develop within the limits of a given situation. The dorsal ascending central nervous system and the ventral descending heart each appear to play a role in the positional development of the nerves and blood vessels within the limb. The ingrowing nerves are situated nearer the brain, i.e. dorsocranially, whereas the ingrowing blood vessels are located nearer the heart, i.e. ventrocaudally. The main arterial paths to both the upper and lower extremities develop ventral and caudal to their respective nerve plexuses. The subclavian artery develops ventrally and caudally to the brachial plexus; the iliac-femoral artery channel develops ventrally and caudally to the lumbosacral plexus.

Nerves converge toward the limb anlage in the same manner as blood vessels and dermatomes. As the nerves make contact with one another at the beginning of the second month they produce plexuses. By the middle of the second month the interior of the shoulder and hip regions contains mostly nerves (cf. 1975, pp. 143, 159). Established nerves and blood vessels consistently grow slower in length than does the tissue in areas of their branches. Because of this phenomenon the nerves and vessels act as restrainers (they have a restraining function). As a result, growth in the length of the early limbs is not rectilinear but instead curves and bends. This is apparent even in the early period of development (Figs. 12-15 and 12-16). These correlations have heretofore never been made.

STRUCTURE OF THE EARLY LIMB ANLAGE

The upper limb bud in a 3.5 mm embryo is composed of only a small number of ectodermal and mesenchymal cells. However, even at this time the main directions of the cells appear to be trajectorial alignments. The flat cells of the periderm are aligned perpendicular to the cells of the stratum basal. The basal cells are arranged as palisades. The cells of the stratum basal as well as the stromal cells are aligned perpendicular to the basement membrane of the ectoderm. The stromal cells near the ectoderm are relatively larger than the deeper mesenchymal cells. Histological sections consistently reveal that many of the basal cells that form strong palisades are covered only by a single peridermal cell. This suggests that the two ectodermal layers develop by way of differing kinetics. The basal layer grows quickly; the periderm grows slowly. The reverse arrangement of the basal layer and periderm has never been found. From the observed morphology it is concluded that the ectodermal cells are polarized. In other words, the ectoderm absorbs nutrients basally and releases waste products (mainly water) peripherally into the amniotic cavity. The polarization promotes the rapid surface area growth of the ectoderm. In contrast to the retarded growth of the periderm, the basal layer of ectoderm appears to grow intensely in surface area caused by the assimilation of nutrients.

The locally different surface growth of the ectoderm causes, by its assimilation, a flow of nutrients in the underlying stroma. As a consequence, the cell multiplication in the stroma becomes locally variable in intensity (development of the corium varies in strength). The intense surface growth of the cutis causes the limb bud to flatten and to form its well-known border. With additional growth the distal border of the limb fold becomes more acute.

It is important to recall at this time the statement that shape and structure are inseparable in the morphological sense. The increased acuteness of the distal limb border is inseparable from the formation of a ridge of ectoderm at the margin of the limb anlage (marginal ridge). Actually, shape and structure are more closely related than are causal correlations. Structure can always be understood as a feature of shape.

The three-dimensional angle under the periderm at the distal border of the limb anlage progressively decreases as the border becomes more acute. The marginal ridge forms as the angle decreases and causes the stratum basal to become more compressed (Fig. 12-7). The arising thickening is very important with regard to the undulating limb border and consequently to the development of the fingers. The marginal ridge develops into three layers (periderm, intermediate stratum and stratum basal). The stratum basal shows long cells, but the intermediate stratum has cubical cells and the periderm shows flattened cells. All available evidence leads to the conclusion that the ridge is a kinetic consequence of the formation of the limb border which, in turn, is a result of limb flattening. There is no proof to support the reverse assumption that limb flattening is caused by the ridge. If the limb anlage did not develop its particular shape, the characteristic acute border would not form. Without such a border, the marginal ridge would be absent.

In accordance with the statement that there are normally no functionless organs, one would expect the marginal ridge to be constructively important for subsequent differentiations. Indeed,

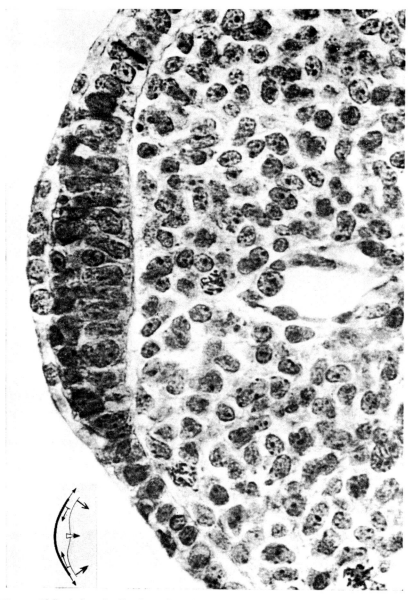

Figure 12-7. A longitudinal section through upper limb anlage of an 8 mm embryo, stage 16, mid-sixth week. 840×. Palmar side is at the top. The marginal (thickened ectodermal) ridge results from the sharply bent ectoderm at distal border of the anlage. Notice that ectoderm here is composed of three layers, a deep stratum basal, an outer periderm and between both a layer with spherical cells and dark nuclei. Arrows in the diagram indicate the biokinetics of the ectoderm in the area of the marginal ridge.

the ridge will be shown to have a very important function after additional limb growth takes place and the limb surface has expanded sufficiently. The marginal ridge is the constructive means by which limb rays are formed in the embryo. Prior to discussing this, however, development of the internal structure of the early limb should be given.

As growth adduction of the limb buds occurs the embryonic cutis becomes relatively shorter and thicker on the flexion side than on the extension side (Fig. 12-6). As was mentioned above, the cutis of the early limb anlagen should be viewed as a tube with a core that is under low pressure. This seems to be brought about by increased surface growth along the basement membrane with simultaneous slower growth of the stroma in the interior of the limb. Such a situation in the early stage of development indicates that the amniotic fluid would exert from the outside a stronger pressure on the ectoderm than does the stroma from the inside. In purely physical terms, there would be a positive pressure exerted from the outside. If the stroma of the limb anlage were artificially inflated by injecting fluid, then the internal pressure would overcome the external opposing pressure of the amniotic fluid. As a result, the limb anlage would lose its flat shape, abduct and become spherical. It is certain that thickening of the cutis on the flexion side of the limb anlage (embryonic palm and sole areas) should be interpreted as a manifestation of locally hindered surface growth.

After gaining a deeper appreciation of the biodynamic origin of differentiations it then becomes necessary to understand the principles by which developmental processes occur in the interior of limb. To some investigators the term "mesenchyma" means a structureless tissue interposed between, and bounded by, epithelium. Blechschmidt's studies reveal that mesenchyma (inner embryonic tissue) is not this at all. To the contrary, this tissue exhibits a trajectorial structure that is very regular (Figs. 12-8 to 12-11). Its structure reveals that there is a close kinetic relationship between limiting tissues (epithelium) and inner tissues.

The cell aggregations and cells in the early limbs are primarily oriented in such a way that their directions are either parallel or perpendicular to the surface of the whole limb anlage. Their directions therefore intersect at particular points. The intercellular substance between the limiting membranes is relatively liquid. In accordance with the findings discussed previously, intercellular substance functions as a site of biomechanical pressure. However, cell limiting membranes are sites of pull. It is most likely that this living push-pull system is what directs metabolism and causes the young limb to have a stable shape even when it represents only a small fraction of the embryonic cutis. This stability can be demonstrated by micromanipulation.

The following generalization is based on observations of numerous microscopic preparations. Consistently, the anlagen of living beings not only have a shape that is related to their position but also retain their shape according to their position. The quality that developing organs have of keeping their shape is an action

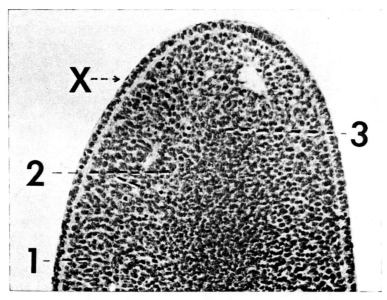

Figure 12-8. A longitudinal section through the upper limb anlage of a 14 mm embryo. 200×. *1*, anlage of dermis where cells are mainly aligned perpendicular to overlying ectoderm; *2*, anlage of subcutis that is very vascular; *3*, distal end of skeleton anlage that is still precartilaginous. Near "X" are the flat nuclei of peridermal cells.

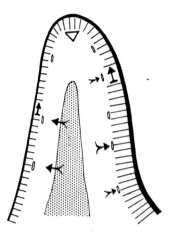

Figure 12-9. Diagram of a longitudinal section through the hand plate of a 15 mm embryo showing the appearance of the tissue layering. Heavy black line represents the ectoderm. Dermis (corium) is hatched, subcutis is white. Densation field for the arising skeleton is stippled. Arrows with base line show surface growth of the cutis. Tailed arrows indicate that densation is an effect of releasing fluid towards the blood vessels (ovals).

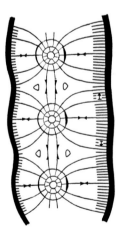

Figure 12-10. Diagram of a transverse section through the hand plate of a 10 mm embryo showing main alignment of the cell limiting membranes. Palm is on right side. Densation fields of precartilage are represented by circles. Arrows indicate same as in previous figures.

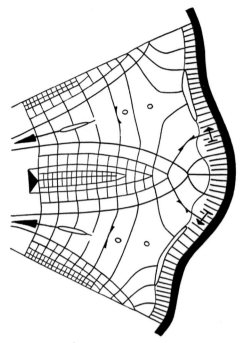

Figure 12-11. Diagram of a frontal section through the hand plate of a 13.5 mm embryo showing main alignments of the mesenchyma. Densation fields in thick portions of plate are represented by narrow meshes. Arrowhead indicates direction of pressure from expanding cartilage. Convergent arrows show restraining action; divergent arrows show direction of increased growth along the limb border. Simple arrows indicate growth pull of blood vessels in the subcutis.

not only of the organ but of the total embryo. In short, even the earliest anlagen of organs already have functional shapes and consequently act as being differentiated (functional differentiation).

Figures 12-9 to 12-11 show the main orientations of the inner tissue of the upper limb anlage on longitudinal, transverse and frontal sections, respectively. These drawings show the main trajectories of the peripheral part of the inner tissue which are primarily aligned perpendicular to the basement membrane of the ectoderm. Where the ectoderm is thick, this layer of inner tissue is also thick. Where the ectoderm is thin, the layer is correspondingly thin. From this, it is obvious that the superficial, dense layer of mesenchyma immediately beneath the ectoderm has a particularly close constructive relationship to the overlying ectoderm. The authors consider this cell aggregation of the inner tissue to be the embryonic dermis (corium) (Fig. 12-8, zone *1*). The dermis together with the embryonic epidermis (ectoderm layer) form a closely connected, unit structure called the embryonic cutis. The cells beneath the dermis layer are more slender and form the early subcutis layer (zone *2*). The subcutis layer contains a relatively large amount of liquid intercellular substance and appears loose.

It is in the subcutis that vascularization develops. This means the ectoderm is not supplied directly by blood vessels but is indirectly provided for by corium cells (Figs. 12-8 and 12-9). The communicating interstices are oriented primarily in the proximo-distal direction. The intercellular substance prepares the area for blood vessels growing distalward. The principle of blood vessel formation was explained previously (Chapter 8). As is the case with all blood vessels, these vessels also act as restrainers after they have grown sufficiently.

The cells deep in the interior of the paddle-shaped appendage show no particular orientation and are mainly spherical (Fig. 12-9, stippled zone). Because of this shape they are especially capable of proliferation. As a result of proliferation, these cells become very crowded thereby forming a characteristic dense area in the inner tissue. Such a dense area is referred to as a *densation field* (this will be discussed further in Chapter 14).

Once again, it may be seen that the limiting tissue of limbs (ectoderm) is polarized like all other limiting tissues. It assimilates nourishment from a single given source on its basal side and releases katabolic waste products, especially water, outwardly into the amniotic cavity. This conclusion has been arrived at partly because no intercellular substance is congested between the ectodermal cells and partly because the volume of amniotic fluid increases as development proceeds. Regional comparisons indicate that the prime intense surface growth activity of the ectoderm is attributable to its ability to release katabolic water into the amniotic cavity.

Blood vessels first become apparent in the embryonic subcutis (Fig. 12-8, zone *2*) rather than in the embryonic dermis (zone *1*). This leads one to assume that nourishment of the ectoderm takes place through the embryonic dermis in a manner that is primarily perpendicular to the basement membrane of the ectoderm. The cells in the metabolic field of the embryonic dermis multiply and grow intensely only near the ectoderm. This indicates that they take in substances from the nourishment which pass to the ectoderm and release waste products into the embryonic subcutis (thereby forming intercellular substance) rather than into the ectoderm. This leads to the formation of venous channels in the early subcutis along with the arteries. Only a kinetic process like this could explain why inner tissue grows faster peripherally than it does in the interior of the limb anlage. This directed kinetic process also explains why the cells of the dermis anlage compress each other into becoming aligned perpendicular to the basement membrane. Because of their alignment the early dermal cells become morphologically similar to epithelial cells.

Differentiation of the skeleton takes place in a special metabolic field and will be described in subsequent chapters.

FAN-LIKE SPREADING MOVEMENTS OF THE LIMB PLATE

It was shown above that the limb fold moves in such a way that it covers over the limb placode. It was also shown how the acute border of the limb anlage arises as a result rather than as a cause of this developmental movement. When the upper limb anlage has the shape of a fold, its cranial end (future shoulder region) is thicker while its caudal end (future elbow region) is thinner (Fig. 12-12, near *1* and *2*). The cranial and caudal ends differ in shape having developed in accordance with the shape of the deeper neural tube–serosa angle, which opens and is wider cranially. The same is true for the lower limb, the neural tube–serosa angle opens and is wider caudally. Consequently the caudal end of the lower limb (future gluteal region) is thicker than the future knee region. Growth of the wedge-shaped epithelium of the ectodermal marginal ridge of the limbs in conjunction with the growth resistance of the underlying stroma would lead to bending of the limb border (Fig. 12-12, first and second diagrams). Bending would be more distinct in the distal part of the limb anlage where the border is more acute. The more acute thin border grows faster than the less acute thick border because its wedge-shaped epithelial cells are more divergent. Thus, an early lanceolate shape appears.

The increasing distal growth causes the formation of the radiate limb rays. The cell limiting membranes and, accordingly, the main lines of tension converge proximally beneath the apex of the distal bend (Fig. 12-12, near 3). Because the cells in the convergence zone are under equal growth tension, their cell bodies become spherical and they undergo mitoses. Proliferation of these cells produces a mesenchymal densation which, in this instance, is the anlage of a skeletal part, the ulna (Fig. 12-12, third and fourth top illustrations). The continued lengthening growth and the subsequent bending of the marginal ridge give rise in the same manner to the anlage of the radius (darkly stippled areas in bottom illustrations). Wherever the marginal ridge of the limb plate bends convexly distalwards, the underlying stroma is compressed. It yields to the narrowing and thickens in the plane transverse to the bend plane forming cell proliferation zones which are the anlagen of the limb rays. With this development, the limb anlage attains a radiating fan-like appearance. The entire margin becomes undulant. Thus, the outer shape of the limb plate determines what structure is established internally (Fig. 12-12). Shape and structure are much more closely related than are cause and effect.

The decisive bendings of the marginal ridge are established as a result of the lengthening of the entire complex of the ectodermal marginal ridge with its connected embryonic dermis. This complex lengthens at a more rapid rate than does the underlying stroma. The outlined distal border of the limb plate indicates this growth in Figures 12-12 and 12-15. The longitudinal growth of the embryonic stroma is retarded in comparison to the intense superficial growth of the embryonic cutis particularly at its distal end. This means that the stroma which is retarded in growth becomes straightened particularly along the quickly growing

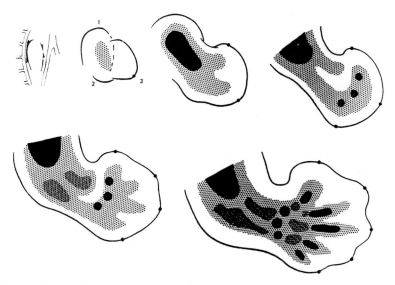

Figure 12-12. Biodynamic relationships between shape and structure of upper limb anlage. Appearance of skeleton anlage in the interior in correlation with growing embryonic cutis (outline). From top left to bottom right, limb anlagen are from embryos approximately 4 mm, 6 mm, 7 mm, 8 mm, 9 mm, and 11mm, respectively. The pisiform carpal bone is not shown as it develops subsequently as a sesamoid bone within a tendon. Drawings are incomplete since ingrowing blood vessels and nerves that exert an important restraining action are not shown. *1,* shoulder area; *2,* elbow area; *3,* forearm area. (For details *see text).*

marginal ridge. As a result of this restriction, the distal ends of the still soft ulna and radius anlagen become more convergent instead of taking their earlier divergent direction. By this movement the distal converging ends of the skeletal anlagen appear to form articulation clefts by becoming sheared off.

Additional segments of the skeleton anlage form as additional bendings develop in the embryonic cutis. The skeletal anlagen multiply one step at a time (Fig. 12-12). After the ulna and radius are established, subsequent bendings cause the formation of three proximal carpal anlagen, then four distal carpal anlagen followed by five metacarpal anlagen. The wavy crests of the marginal ridge that form the epithelial anlage of the digits only develop after the appearance of the metacarpal anlagen, never before. They occur approximately in the middle of the second month.

It is during the second month that differentiation is greatest. During this time period, rhythmic deformations of the limb anlage become visible. They are caused by vascular pulsation. The embryonic dermis appears to be stretched circularly by each vascular pulsation, mainly in the limb stalk that is developing proximal to the limb plate. The structure of the embryonic dermis in this area is aligned in a circular fashion related to the longitudinal path of the arteries, i.e. circular to the longitudinal axis of the extremity. The alignment appears to be the result of vascular pulsations. Since the limb stalk is reinforced by the circularly structured embryonic dermis, its length increases more rapidly than does its circumference. The digits later show a similar longitudinal growth.

Lengthening of the limb anlage does not occur rectilinearly.

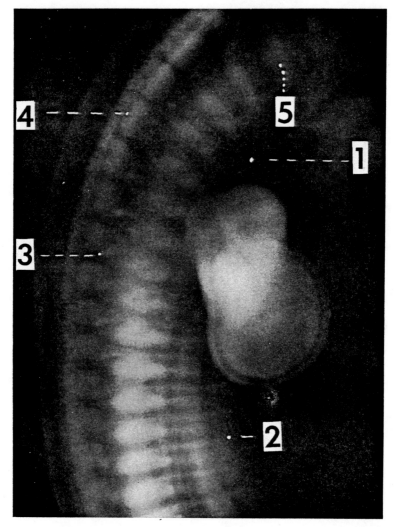

Figure 12-13. Lateral view of upper limb anlage of an 8.8 mm embryo. 30×.
1, region of the common cardinal vein; *2*, ventral branch of the T7 spinal
nerve; *3*, lateral branch of the T1 spinal nerve; *4*, exit of the dorsal root of
the C6 spinal ganglion; *5*, intervertebral disc.

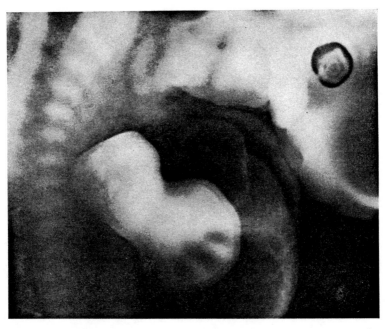

Figure 12-14. Lateral view of upper limb anlage of an 11.1 mm embryo, stage 17, end of the sixth week. 20×. Thick parts of anlage appear light. Limb rays of metacarpus are alternately light (thick zones) and dark (thin zones). Marginal ridge is grey zone at periphery of hand plate.

Stems of particularly large vascular channels form on the flexion side of the limb anlage in accordance with the thickening of the embryonic subcutis in this region. These vessels remain relatively short in comparison to the cell aggregations they supply (Fig. 12-16.) In this manner they assist in the development of the growth flexion of the digits. Growth flexion becomes more intense because of the growth resistance of the very strong flexor tendon anlage. After several weeks all of the digit anlagen are flexed approximately 180° except those of the thumb and the big toe which are flexed only 90°. During these developmental movements the most acutely bent digits differentiate into three segments, i.e. proximal, intermediate and distal, whereas the less acutely bent thumb and big toe differentiate into only two segments.

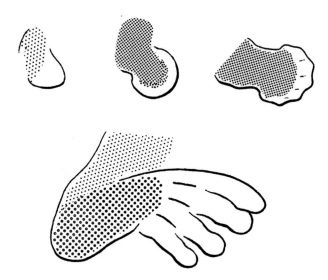

Figure 12-15. Upper limb anlage from 6.3 mm, 10 mm, 13 mm and 29 mm embryos. Drawings show lateral and ventral aspects with arm, forearm and carpus areas stippled. White zones at periphery are sites of appositional growth. Growth grasping movement during development can be appreciated by rapidly viewing the drawings in series.

GROWTH GRASPING AND KICKING MOVEMENTS OF THE LIMBS

During early growth adduction of the upper and lower limb anlagen, the hepatic bulge and umbilical cord, respectively, are situated adjacent to them. These positional relationships are important in the further determination of limb development. In accordance with the increasing restraining function of the vessels and nerves, the upper limb anlage bends progressively more in the elbow area and the hand area moves cranialward over the heart bulge. As this movement occurs, the forearm segment gradually undergoes pronation.

Simultaneous with the developmental movements in the upper limb are growth movements in the lower limb that resemble kicking. It is difficult to determine what are walking, sitting or standing growth movements. However, as development proceeds the embryonic heel treads more and more in the angle between

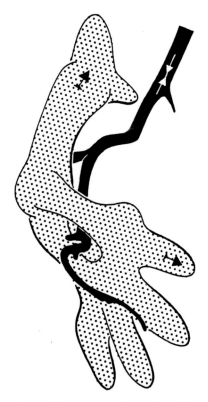

Figure 12-16. Part of a serial reconstruction of a 10 mm embryo showing skeletal and arterial anlagen in the upper limb. Divergent arrows in the skeletal anlage represent the distusion directions of cartilage. Convergent arrows in arterial anlage show its restraining function. As a result, growth flexion occurs in elbow area before joint appears.

the lower abdominal wall and the umbilical cord. This causes dorsiflexion of the foot before the ankle joint forms.

The nervous system also participates in limb development during the second month. The participation of nerves appears earlier in the upper limb than in the lower limb because the former has a closer relationship to the rapidly growing brain and, thus, was innervated earlier. Information on the growth movements of the early developed upper limb is transmitted to the brain at a particularly early time.

SECTION II

LATE METABOLIC FIELDS

Whereas the previous section deals with the kinetics of early differentiations, Section II contains applications of the kinetic theory to later differentiations. This section presents these differentiations with regard to the characteristics of their metabolic fields. The histochemical and biochemical changes that accompany differentiations are outside the scope of this monograph. Indeed, such investigations fall short of generally describing the standard features of differentiation processes or the orderly manner in which they occur.

The position, shape and structure of metabolic fields during the later developmental stages undergo changes from one moment to another. These changes are always changes of the outward appearance of the entire organism. Whatever is constant during the changing developmental stages, under normal conditions, is the intrinsic nature of any living thing. The intrinsic nature with the help of metabolism, is what causes individuality. This section will present main directions of the developmental movements and describe the kinetics of the development. The general rules of differentiation that are applicable to man very likely have much in common with the rules of the developmental movements that take place in animals and even in plants. Unfortunately, a complete series of embryonic animal and plant specimens comparable to those of man are not yet available. Comparisons between the features of human and animal development are not

181

possible until precisely staged series are available. A series of total reconstructions would be required. If this were done, it would then be possible to determine the developmental kinetic processes that any given animal has in common with man. Since such series of reconstructions are not yet available, comments must be restricted to the human situation.

13

CORROSION FIELDS

In Chapter 2 it was shown how important the reduction in the volume of cells, e.g. blastomeres is to later developmental constructions of the ovum. The process of cell volume reduction may be so great that it results in the total disappearance of the cells. Such an event particularly occurs in *corrosion fields*. A corrosion field is established when two epithelial layers are pressed together to form a thin, double-layered membrane. This is a consistent finding and a fundamental rule for this type of metabolic field (Fig. 13-1). In a corrosion field the adjoining cells undergo necrosis at varying speeds thereby causing a defect in the tissue. It is in this manner that communications are established either between fluids or sometimes between inner tissues that are adjacent to the two epithelial layers.

Limiting tissues (epithelia) are sufficiently nourished during development only through the underlying inner tissue. They release waste products into the adjacent fluids. In other words, there is a metabolic gradient between inner tissue and fluid. This implicates epithelia as being diathelia. This concept was presented in Chapter 3. Studies on the corrosion of membrane-like, double-layered cell aggregations lend support to this concept. When the supporting inner tissue or the fluid between the two epithelial layers disappears, the metabolic gradient of the epithelia

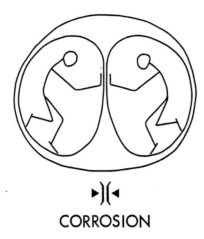

▶)(◀

CORROSION

Figure 13-1. A simplified demonstration of the kinetic movements associated with a corrosion field. The two "matchstick men" press two walls strongly against each other. At the site of contact the wall materials perish giving rise to a perforation. When the limiting tissues (epithelia) are compressed so closely that there is no remaining space for vascularized inner tissue, then the supply ceases and the cells undergo necrosis. Metabolic fields in which epithelial cells perish in such a manner are referred to as corrosion fields.

becomes reduced and the epithelia lose their diathelial ability. When this occurs, the normal conditions for nourishment of the epithelial cells are absent. An adequate supply to the epithelia is no longer possible. This can be seen by necrosis of the epithelial cells. The area in which necrosis occurs is referred to as a corrosion field.

As the vitality of the two-layered epithelia decreases and the adjacent tissue which borders the epithelia undergoes growth, the membrane-like cell aggregation ruptures in the metabolic field that has become insufficient for adequate nourishment of the epithelial cells. Blechschmidt (1961) pointed out and described such rupture zones in a large number of areas in the embryo. A survey and some of the consequences of such corrosion fields will be given here.

Of the many corrosion fields that occur during development the following are given as examples. During the second week of development such a field is present in the contact area between the axial process and the underlying endoderm (Figs. 4-4 and 4-5). Examples of corrosion fields in the developing urogenital system are the contact areas between the mesonephric tubules and mesonephric duct, as well as between the nephrons and the branches of the ureteric tree; between the two layers of the cloacal membrane; and between the seminiferous tubules and the rete testis.

In the head region there are many corrosion fields such as the contact area between the two-layered oropharyngeal (buccopharyngeal) membrane that separates the amniotic and foregut fluids (cf. 1975, p. 33), and between the double-layered oronasal (bucconasal) membrane in the area of the primary choanae (p. 199). A corrosion field with reduced fluid between the epithelial layers is present in the junction region between the palatine processes (p. 275). Another region where fluid is absent is where the neural folds make contact with each other thereby closing the neural groove (p. 45).

Corrosion fields are also observed in developing blood vessels. The medial walls of the paired dorsal aortae make contact when their structure is still similar to that of a capillary (pp. 41, 81). As the vessels approach each other in the midline, their adjoining medial walls break down. The lumina of the vessels thereby communicate. The initially paired ventral spinal arteries also meet and fuse in the midline into one vessel (Figs. 13-2 and 13-3).

The examples mentioned above represent only a small portion of the corrosion fields that actually exist. The many examples show the dynamic nature of differentiation processes. Corrosion fields are so widespread it is surprising that this was not concluded many years ago.

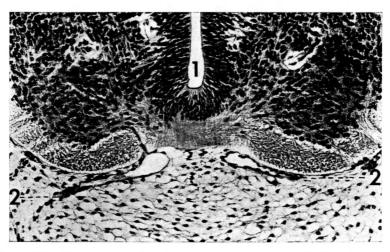

Figure 13-2. Transverse section through the ventral part of the spinal cord of an 11 mm embryo, stage 17, end of 6th week. 200×. A corrosion field develops between the ventral spinal arteries (*2*) that are paired at this stage. *1,* central canal.

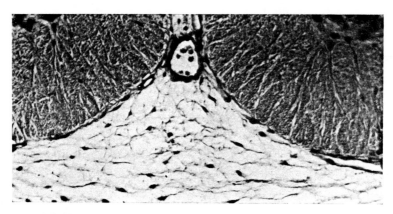

Figure 13-3. Transverse section through the ventral part of the spinal cord of a 28 mm embryo, stage 23, end of second month, 230×. The previously paired ventral spinal artery is now single as a result of the corrosion field where endothelia are compressed against each other with subsequent rupture.

14

DENSATION FIELDS

Biological data are becoming available today
so rapidly that it is difficult to view them as more than a collection
of facts. Serious attempts must be made to interrelate and organ-
ize this abundant new information if the understanding of living
systems is to become more meaningful. For example, differentiation during man's early development should follow a set of rules.
It is very necessary that one seeks to find these rules. What follows
is the attempt to describe conclusively the differentiation of the
arising cartilaginous skeleton. In Blechschmidt's investigations, not
only cartilaginous tissue is considered as belonging to the skeleton
but also the perichondrium, joints, joint capsules and joint ligaments. With this understanding, the following statements are
made only after having compared developmental movements in
different regions.

As is known, the appearance of the skeleton is preceded by
mesenchymal "densations." Such "densations" occur in what is
referred to as a *densation field*. Such a field is a metabolic zone
composed of cells with rather spherical cell bodies and very little
intercellular substance present between the cells. Dense mesenchymal fields differ essentially from loosened ones by the amount
of liquid intercellular substance present. Mesenchymal loosening
zones arise when intercellular liquid moves or is pressed from

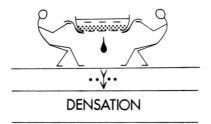

DENSATION

Figure 14-1. Simple demonstration of the kinetic movements associated with a densation field. The matchstick men bear a bowl containing solid and liquid contents. Fluid leaves and consequently the solid particles are brought nearer to each other. The draining of fluid causes a condensation. Metabolic fields in which the positional relationship between cells and liquid components changes in favor of the cells are referred to as densation fields.

surrounding structures into the mesenchyma, e.g. the loosening of the arachnoid as intercellular liquid leaves the brain and spinal cord (cf. 1961, p. 255). On the other hand, movement of intercellular liquid from within the mesenchyma to the periphery causes it to become dense (Fig. 14-1).

The first microscopically distinct anlage of the extremity skeleton is an example of a densation field. Initially, this blastema is rather undifferentiated. Regional comparisons show that only part of the blastema becomes cartilage. Joints, joint capsules and ligaments also arise from the blastema. In light of this, it should be pointed out that the term precartilage is ambiguous and misleading when referring to such a blastema. This term leads one to believe that such areas give rise only to cartilage which is known to be erroneous.

It seems fruitless to try and trace the course of histogenesis from any "preformed" plan in the nucleus. Normal developmental constructions are not initiated genetically from inside the cell but from outside the cell. One must look to the outside for the answer. The biodynamical circumstances in which the mesenchymal skeleton arises should be examined in order to determine the local biodynamic modifications of tissue differentiations. All of the densation fields that were investigated are characterized by their position. Not only is the position of the field itself significant but also the position of the cells and their nuclei. Such a position is always related to the neighboring differentiations. This relationship to neighboring differentiations is very important and is usually overlooked by most investigators.

As an example of how the local biodynamic differentiations of tissue are determined a transverse section through the embryonic trachea may be closely examined (Fig. 14-2). The epithelium on the dorsal side (bottom of figure) of the tracheal anlage is thicker than that on the opposite side. The cells adjacent to the thicker epithelium are elongated and tangentially aligned (1). They will subsequently give rise to the trachealis muscle and fibrous membrane. On the opposite side, the stroma has the appearance of a densation field composed of many closely aggregated cells with rather spherical cell bodies and large nuclei (2). There is little

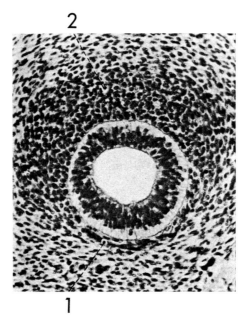

Figure 14-2. Transverse section through the tracheal anlage of an 11 mm embryo, stage 17, end of 6th week. 210×. Shows the appearance of a densation field (2) where tracheal cartilage develops adjacent to the thinner epithelium. The trachealis muscle differentiates in a dilation field (Chapter 18) adjacent to the thicker epithelium (1).

intercellular substance in this zone. The developmental kinetics of this region are explained in Figure 14-3. The thicker epithelium (bottom of figure) appears to grow more rapidly (divergent arrows) than does its counterpart on the opposite side (small convergent arrows). As this occurs, the adjacent stroma is expanded by means of the surface growth of the epithelium causing the cells there to elongate and align tangentially. Opposite to this zone in the stroma there exists a densation field (convergent arrows). The circumstances in this zone are such that the cells which earlier were fairly long because of the surface growth of the epithelium now shorten and become spherical. The spherical cells proliferate and become mainly the prestructure of cartilage.

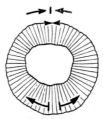

Figure 14-3. Biokinetic explanation of Figure 14-2 based on the developmental movements in the region of the embryonic trachea.

As is known, the trachea is composed of many individual cartilages rather than a single, continuous cartilaginous plate. The biomechanics of this development explains how this configuration forms. In an earlier report, it was stated that as the tracheal anlage lengthens caudalward, the ventral epithelium is thrown into small undulating folds (cf. 1961, p. 395). The cells of the undulating epithelium become wedge-shaped. The limiting membranes of its cells alternately converge and diverge toward the stroma along the undulation. The mesenchyma adjacent to the converging epithelial cells is hindered in space and, therefore, becomes condensed. Subsequently, each of the condensed areas of the stroma differentiates into a contusion field (Chapter 15) thereby forming a tracheal cartilage.

The biokinetic principle of a densation field is also valid for other formations, for example, the early differentiation of the ribs.

The developing thoracic region expands when the heart-liver mass increases. As this mass enlarges, the mesenchymal tissue between the spinal nerves in the thoracic wall is initially stretched in a curved manner at the periphery of the mass. As the heart-liver mass continues to expand, the stretched tissue becomes less curved or, in other words, straightens. This means that the former elongated cells become spherical. Here again, densation fields are established at the outer aspect of the stretched tissue areas and give rise to the rib anlagen (Fig. 11-2).

Another example of a densation field is the developing area adjacent to the basal or ventral part of the dura mater anlage or brain capsule. The basal portion is initially very curved. As the developing brain expands eccentrically the basal part of its capsule is straightened relative to its previously curved configuration. A mesenchymal densation field appears at the periphery of the capsule as the latter structure straightens (Fig. 14-4, *1*). The densation field here represents the anlage of the skull base. An analogous finding can be observed at the periphery of the spinal dura mater anlage ventral to the expanding spinal cord (Fig. 9-5).

A densation field is also observed during differentiation of the

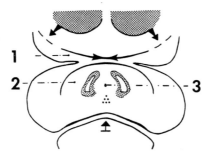

Figure 14-4. Taken from a section through the superficial face of a 17 mm embryo showing some of the biokinetic movements in this region. Uppermost arrows show the growth expansion of the cerebral hemispheres. Lower arrow indicates growth expansion of the heart. Convergent arrows represent the restraining function of the embryonic dura mater (brain capsule). The nasal epithelium (oval-like stippled areas) undergoes surface growth. *1, 2,* location of densation fields; *3,* densation field (nasal septum) with stippled triangular area representing the transversely cut stretched fibers in the lower part of the septum in accordance with Figure 14-5.

nasal septum (Figs. 14-4 and 14-5). It is a characteristic differentiation area. When the embryo bends ventrally into a **C**-shape, the lower free border of the early nasal septum becomes aligned in a manner parallel to the curved dorsum of the tongue (Fig. 14-5, convergent arrows). This converts the free border into a smooth, ventrocaudally directed, concave arch. When the cardiac bulge enlarges *(2),* the nose area becomes pressed against it causing the nose to tilt in an upward direction (upper arrow). This causes the formation of the typical "snub nose" at this particular period (cf. 1977). As a consequence of the nose tilting upward, the nasal septal arch straightens and the epithelial meatuses become narrowed in accordance with the straightening of the septal tissue (Fig. 14-5, *1*).

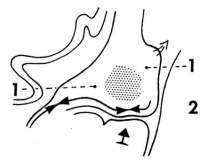

Figure 14-5. Taken from a midsagittal plane through the nasal region of a 20 mm embryo showing some of the biokinetic movements in this area. Densation field (*1*) appears as the snub nose develops (outlined arrow). *2,* cardiac prominence. Convergent arrows in the lower edge of the nasal septum show the restraining function of the stretched mesenchyma in this area. Arrow with base line indicates the growth pressure of the embryonic lower jaw.

At this time, it is necessary to emphasize again that differentiation in a densation field is not mechanical but biomechanical and consequently a biodynamic process requiring the metabolism of the living cells. A particularly important feature of a characteristic densation field is that it is established in zones where the cells have mainly elongated shapes at the time of their deformation into becoming spherical. The cells in densation fields show no particular orientation. This means that they are under a tension stress which is equal in all directions and, consequently, they become spherical. The cell-crowded mesenchymal area expanding by growth and adjacent to epithelia are referred to in Chapter 15.

15

CONTUSION FIELDS

W HEN A DENSATION field transforms into cartilage
the spherical cells that compose it, first gradually undergo flattening. This flattening normally occurs in a radial plane around
the longitudinal axis of the densation focus. Initially, zones of
flattened cells are found only in the center of an enlarged densation field that has attained sufficient size. The cells in this region
of the densed mesenchyma develop into cartilage cells thereby
forming a focus of young cartilage. Such a metabolic field is referred to as a *contusion field*.

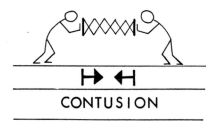

Figure 15-1. Simple demonstration of the kinetic movements associated with
a contusion field. Two matchstick men are compressing a spring. As the
spring shortens in one dimension, it widens in the other. Similarly, when
spherical mesenchymal cells become compressed from two opposing directions (convergent pressure arrows) they flatten and become disc-shaped.
Such compression zones give rise to young cartilage and are referred to as
contusion fields.

Investigations by Blechschmidt show that flattening of the spherical cells in a densation field is a prerequisite for their subsequent transformation into cartilage cells. Here is yet another example of a structural predevelopment that is necessary for subsequent differentiations to occur. Such a predevelopment can be shown to be directed from the outside inward rather than from the inside outward.

Contusion fields are always surrounded by a perichondrium which merges with the surrounding loose mesenchyma. A good example of this feature is the formation of the supporting structure of the nasal conchae (cf. 1961, p. 337).

The terms "densation field" and "contusion field" are sometimes confused. Densation field refers to a condensation zone that is made up of spherical cells. On the other hand, a contusion field refers to a compression zone where the cells become flattened. A representation of the general biodynamic features of a contusion field is shown in Figure 15-1. The spring represents the spherical cells in a densation field that are being compressed on two sides. As compression develops, the spring narrows in the longitudinal plane and simultaneously widens in the plane perpendicular to the longitudinal axis. Similarly, spherical cells flatten and become disc-shaped in a plane perpendicular and radial to the longitudinal axis.

The kinetic principles of a contusion field can be understood by closely examining regions where cartilaginous structures differentiate. Generally, the kinetic features of a densation field can be observed in the differentiation of the skeletal anlage in limb buds. Where the skeleton arises, the cells within a limb underneath the subcutis always initially exhibit almost equal cell diameters in all three dimensions. In other words, they generally have a spherical shape. The epithelium which encloses these cells provides the condition for the densation (Fig. 12-8). At the distal end of the limb buds, when they each have the shape of a fold, cell limiting membranes cross one another in the three dimensions. Such an arrangement implies that growth tensions of near equal intensity are equally distributed. It is precisely in the region where such trajectories cross that one finds cells with equal

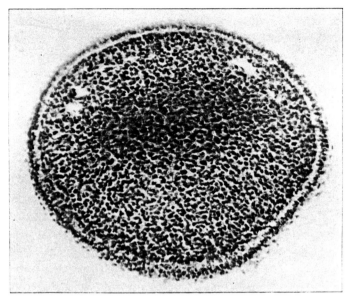

Figure 15-2. Transverse section through the finger end of a 17 mm embryo. 200×. The condensation in the interior of the finger is a densation field. It is eccentrically located and represents the skeletal anlage. The position of the condensation coincides with the zone where radially arranged surface trajectories intersect one another (*see* Figure 15-3). The peripheral cell-dense zone beneath the ectoderm is the dermis anlage. The loose tissue between the two dense zones contains more abundant intercellular liquid and vascular channels (subcutis anlage).

spatial dimensions. Such cells consequently have a spherical shape (Figs. 15-2 and 15-3).

Contusion fields with typical disc-like, broad, flat cells form within such zones of condensation or densation fields. The cells flatten in the direction of least resistance, i.e. transverse to the longitudinal axis of the limbs. These findings strongly suggest that the trajectorial structure of the mesenchyma in embryonic limbs is very important in the construction and formation of the cartilaginous skeleton.

The biodynamic uniformity of these differentiations can be appreciated by the examination of a transverse section through the finger end of a 17 mm embryo's limb. The densation field in

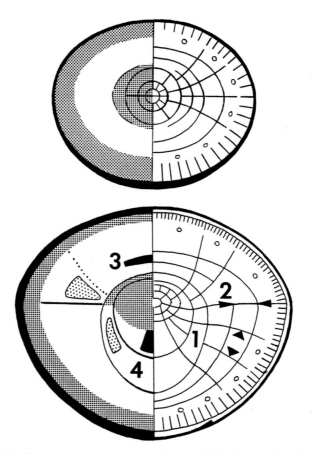

Figures 15-3. Transverse sections through a middle finger of a 17 mm embryo at various levels showing diagrammatically the main alignments of the mesenchymal meshes. Densation fields (corium and precartilage) are stippled. *1*, symmetric site of the great ventral conduction pathways (stipple); *2*, symmetric site of the great dorsal conduction pathways (stipple); *3*, site of the dorsal subcutis; *4*, site of the ventral subcutis. Black areas represent the dorsal aponeurosis and the flexor tendon, respectively. Arrows show biodynamic pull and pressure tensions. The small circles indicate the vascularization beneath the cutis.

the interior represents the anlage of the skeleton (Fig. 15-3). The zone of densation (the skeletal anlage) is characterized by little or no intercellular substances and by cells with no growth tension in any special direction and which have consequently become round. They multiply and subsequently grow resorbing nutrients from the intercellular substance and thereby attract each other and squeeze the fluid intercellular substance towards the periphery. Here, the densation was established by loss of the liquid intercellular substance.

In contrast, the peripheral condensed zone just beneath the epithelium (the anlage of the dermis or corium) becomes dense because of cell multiplication as many mitotic figures are evident. In the dermis anlage the cells are closely packed near the epithelium which are supplied together with nutrients. As a result of their growth they expand and therefore suppress each other and align perpendicular against the basement membrane. The mesenchyma between the inner, cell-crowded densation field and the outer, cell-crowded dermis zone becomes loosened by the accumulation of liquid intercellular substance. Here, the interstices are large. The spatial alignment of the cells indicates a tensile stress that causes the cell volume to be diminished in relation to cell surface. During this process, intracellular liquid becomes intercellular liquid causing the loose appearance of the tissue (Fig. 15-2) where katabolites are accumulated which are released from the neighboring zones and from the vessels with a sufficiently strong pulsating fluid pressure. The arrowheads in Figure 15-3 represent the hydrostatic pressure of the liquid in this zone.

The kinetic factors that bring about the development of precartilage from mesenchyma generally apply with slight modifications for the development of precartilage at the edge of preexisting cartilage in later stages. The zone of such precartilage is also initially composed of closely aggregated elongated cells which subsequently shorten and become spherical (densation field). Growth resistance in one direction gives rise to a contusion field in which the spherical cells flatten and become young cartilage cells. The cells must undergo flattening before dense mesenchyma (spheric-mesenchyma) can transform into cartilage which contains vesicular cells (Chapter 16).

The region of appositional growth of a cartilaginous vertebral arch can be used as an example of the manner in which precartilage at the edge of preexisting cartilage becomes transformed into cartilage (Fig. 15-4). The cartilaginous vertebral arch is growing into the stretched mesenchymal wall of the vertebral canal. The cells making up the stretched wall of the vertebral canal have elongated shapes. They are aligned primarily perpendicular to the direction of the neighboring layers of cartilage cells. Spherical-shaped cells that exhibit frequent mitoses occur between these two orthogonally aligned cell aggregations (Fig. 15-4). A spherical-shaped cell indicates that there is no main

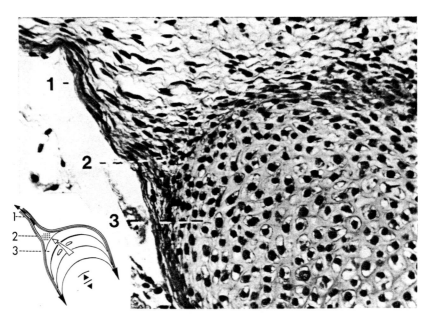

Figures 15-4. Transverse section through a 28 mm embryo at the level of the fourth vertebral arch. 350×. Section shows the transition zone between the arch and its doral continuation with the connective tissue wall of the vertebral canal. Inset at lower left is a diagram of the kinetic movements in this area. *1,* retension field (Chapter 17) with long, straightened cells (arrow in canal wall indicates direction of pull); *2,* densation field with spherical cells attracted to each other by the absorption of nutrients; *3,* contusion field with flattened cells. Outlined arrow shows main growth direction of the cartilaginous vertebral arch. Simple arrows show restraining function of the perichondrum. Triangles represent distusion pressure (Chapter 16) as the flattened cells become vesicular.

growth pull on it and consequently it has no main orientation. As growth proceeds, these cells flatten as an adaptation to the expanding cartilage which increases in volume. This flattening then gives the cells the ability to form cartilage (Chapter 16).

The end of the cartilaginous vertebral arch grows progressively into the fibrous (desmal) wall of the vertebral canal that is stretched by the enlarging spinal cord. The growing arch uses the fibrous wall as a guiding structure. Here again is an example of a differentiation that takes place within a growth functional system. Analogous framing processes were observed in all of the sufficiently early cartilaginous centers that were studied. Nothing has been found that is incompatible with the statement that cartilage development proceeds according to growth functional principles.

In summary, precartilaginous densation fields generally occur where mesenchymal cells become spherical (tension is equally distributed in all directions), multiply, enlarge and squeeze or press out the liquid intercellular substances attracting each other by resorbing the nutrients that are present between them. These factors give rise to specific tissue densations. Contusion fields develop in the interior of a densation field when there is resistance in the longitudinal axis to the growing spherical cells. This growth resistance causes compression (Fig. 15-1) which in turn, causes the cells to flatten thereby transforming them into disc-shaped, young cartilage cells.

16

DISTUSION FIELDS

As with any theory, a theory of development requires that a synopsis be made of the collected data. As a result of such a general review new conclusions may be reached which could not have been determined from the study of isolated facts alone. The discourse that follows on the development of cartilage in distusion fields is based on such a review. A simplified example of the developmental movements that occur in these fields is shown in Figure 16-1.

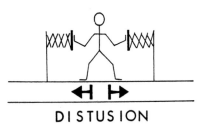

DISTUSION

Figure 16-1. Simplified demonstration of the developmental movements associated with a distusion field. A matchstick man firmly plants each arm against a spring. As the matchstick man pushes in an outward direction or "distuses", the springs yield. This process is referred to as a distusion function (Stemmkörperfunktion). Aggregations of cartilage cells which swell while absorbing fluid, press in a similar manner. Their distusion function exerts pressure on the neighboring tissue (divergent pressure arrows). Zones of cartilage that expand by swelling growth in one main direction are referred to as distusion fields.

Examination of the limbs of a two-month embryo reveals that the older cartilage is located in the proximal portion of the limbs while the younger cartilage is located distally. In addition, cartilage appears first in the central rather than the peripheral part of precartilage that has become sufficiently thick. This positional relationship of the centers of arising cartilage implies that the precartilage cells, which first transform into cartilage cells, are those that are located the greatest distance from the surrounding vascularized mesenchyma.

A clearer understanding of the process of cartilage development can be gained by closely examining the differentiation of a phalanx and using it as an example. Near the growing tip of the embryonic finger the previously spherical cells appear to yield to the growth pressure of the neighboring cells, thereby causing them to broaden perpendicular to the longitudinal axis of the phalanx. As a result, the spherical cells become flattened or disc-shaped (Fig. 16-2, young cartilage with flattened cells in a contusion field). The disc-shaped cells then become vesicular-shaped by increasing in volume. Changes in the position, shape and structure of young cartilage cells are in accordance with changes in their volume and occur in the following manner.

The plate-like, disc-shaped young cartilage cells are located in a metabolic field that seems to have lost much of its permeability. That is, there seems to be a decrease in the importation of nutritive substances as well as in the removal of katabolic waste products. Direct supply and drainage by blood vessels is absent. The cells exhibit very high osmolarity. The high osmolarity of living cartilage has been verified and quantitated by measuring its freezing point. The flattened, highly osmolar cells (contusion field) resorb water from their immediate environment and become vesicular-shaped thereby forming cartilage (distusion field). As water is resorbed from the surrounding tissue, the latter seems to be more solid and fibrils of the ground substance surrounding each cell appear stretched.

The dimensions of the cells change as they go from disc-shape to spherical-shape. This causes the cartilaginous cell mass to grow primarily in one axis (Figs. 16-4 and 16-5, divergent arrows). Because

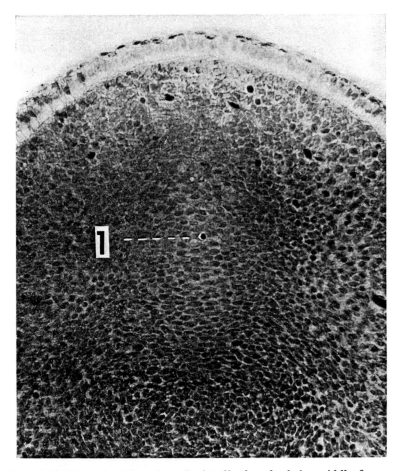

Figure 16-2. Frontal section through the distal end of the middle finger of an 18 mm embryo, stage 20, 8th week. 330×. A young distusion field is located in the zone of the distal phalanx anlage (*1*).

this type of growth is actually a swelling phenomenon, metabolic fields with such metabolic movements are referred to as *distusion fields* (Fig. 16-1). The swelling growth in such fields is parallel to the long axis of the previous precartilaginous skeletal part. Such cartilage growth has a piston (distusion) action (Stemmkörperfunktion) in relation to its surrounding tissue environment.

The distusion function of differentiating cartilage is evident by the fact that the mesenchyma adjacent to the diaphysis is stretched parallel to the main growth direction of the cartilage. Examination of the perichondrium reveals that it is generally stretched longitudinally.

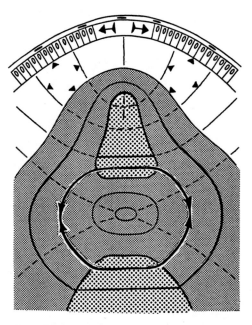

Figure 16-3. Drawing of the section in Figure 16-2 showing its developmental kinetics. Large stippling represents cartilage zones, fine stipple shows location of cell-crowded mesenchyma. Divergent arrows in ectoderm indicate surface growth. Arrowheads represent pressure of the intercellular fluid in the subcutis zone. The restraining function of the collateral ligament anlagen is shown by converging arrows. The interrupted lines represent continuation of pull-tensions of the cutis.

As the quantity of water increases in the large vesicular cartilage cells an opposite process takes place in the surrounding ground substance, i.e. the water content decreases with a resultant hardening to form a capsule around the cells. The movement of water from the ground substance is so intense that its gradual calcification becomes distinct. Here is another example of the

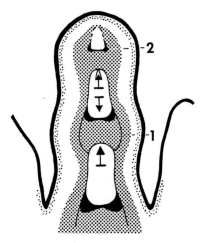

Figure 16-4. Drawing of the same section as in Figure 16-2 but including also the proximal part of the middle finger. Arrows with base line indicate the distusion function of the cartilaginous anlagen of the phalanx. *1,* joint capsule anlage; *2,* level of the apex of the distal articulation loop.

close spatial relationship that exists between neighboring differentiations. Hardening of the calcification zones is an important condition for subsequent bone development (Chapter 20).

Because of its distusion growth the cartilaginous skeleton is the first active part of the locomotor or "mover" apparatus within the embryo. Distusion movements are constructive prerequisites for the origin of so-called articulation loops which will be described below using the interphalangeal joints as examples.

It was shown previously (Chapter 12) that as growth of the upper limb anlage occurs, the limb undergoes adduction. It was also shown that, as growth adduction takes place, surface growth of the ectoderm on the volar (palmar) side of the anlage appears to be hindered and consequently, it thickens. Biodynamically related to this differentiation is the formation of vascular channels (arteries) that occur mainly in the subcutis anlage on the volar side. The subcutis anlage is also thicker on the volar side than on the dorsal side of the limb. The earlier formation of arterial channels on the volar side is a plausible cause of the early growth

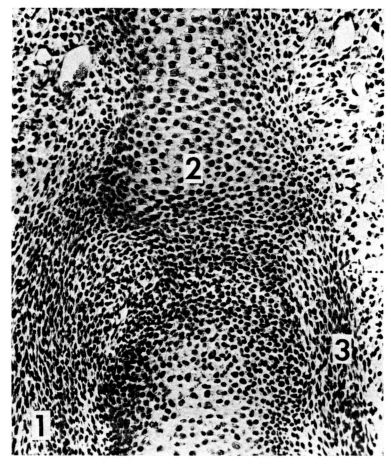

Figure 16-5. Sagittal section through the distal interphalangeal joint of a 27.2 mm embryo, stage 22, end of second month. 250×. The flexor *(1)* and extensor *(3)* portions of the articulation loop are shown. *2,* apex of the loop.

flexion of the fingers since it was shown previously that blood vessels act as restrainers (exhibit restraining functions).

Following the flattening of the finger anlage, which is a result of surface growth, the mesenchymal tissue between the cartilaginous skeleton (anlage of the phalanges) and the cutis anlage is consistently stretched in a longitudinal manner on both the volar and dorsal sides (Fig. 16-5). This tissue stretching is caused by the swelling growth of the cartilage and subsequently is formed as tendons that are aligned in the direction of the distusion (longitudinally). The stretched tissue on the volar and dorsal sides of the cartilaginous phalanx are continuous with each other distal to the end of the phalanx. Such a connection is referred to as an *articulation loop*. However, a joint capsule is not formed. It becomes established only in skeletal regions where the tissue is stretched in two dimensions. This occurs because of the broadening of the joint head in later stages. Articulation loops appear in the proximal part of the limb earlier and are therefore older than the more distal loops. Since the volar segment of the loop has become thicker and stronger than the dorsal segment in accordance with the growth adduction of limb, it gradually gives more resistance to the distusion growth of the phalanx. When the cartilaginous phalanx attains the appropriate length, the growth resistance of the dorsal and volar segments of the articulation loop is so unequal that it causes the tissue on the concave side of the articulation loop to come apart or shear. This tissue shearing in the skeleton anlage is so severe that a tissue gap is formed which represents the joint anlage. The joint gaps make their appearance gradually during this growth luxation of the tissue. The dislocation is aligned in the dorsovolar plane in accordance with the stronger growth resistance of the flexor anlage. (Fig. 17-7).

The tip of the developing finger does not have a symmetrical circular form on transverse section but, being a continuation of the flat hand plate is broader in the radioulnar (lateromedial) plane than in the dorsovolar plane. In other words, the finger tip is oval on transverse section rather than circular (Fig. 15-3). Because of this configuration, when the developing finger tip tilts volarward following the main growth pull of the articulation loops, the radioulnar diameter increases to a greater extent than the dorsovolar diameter. The epiphyseal portion of the phalanx anlage becomes broader in the radioulnar direction in accordance with this phenomenon. Besides the locomotor apparatus there are other examples of broadening as a result of bending, e.g. cranial neuropore with the resulting optic sulci and folds in the early lower head region with the resulting pharyngeal arches.

Broadening of the epiphysis as the fingers undergo growth flexion causes the joint capsule to appear and to be stretched bilaterally, thereby forming the collateral ligaments (Fig. 16-4). The collateral ligaments act as reinforcement bands when joint capsules have been stretched and have a restraining function (Fig. 16-3, converging arrows). Throughout Blechschmidt's investigations there has never been found an exception to the statement that *even in embryonic development all ligaments act as restrainers, i.e. function as restraining structures.* It is unfortunate that ligament development has received little attention. If one refers to the standard handbooks in embryology one would come away

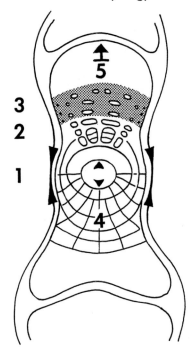

Figure 16-6. Drawing of a section through the intermediate phalanx of a 59 mm fetus. Convergent arrows show the resistance or pull of the surface membrane ("periosteum") that hinders the growing trajectorial system of the cell aggregations. Arrowheads in the center of the phalanx show the expansion force of the vesicular cartilage. Top arrow represents the distusion function of the cartilage (Stemmkörperfunktion). *1,* level of vesicular cartilage; *2,* level of columnar cartilage; *3,* level of cartilage with flat cells and much intercellular material; *4,* metaphysis; *5,* epiphysis.

with the idea that ligaments do not develop at all.

When water accumulates in the osmolar cartilage cells and the cell aggregations in the early diaphysis enlarge sufficiently, the cartilage foci change into long cartilage (Figs. 16-6 and 16-7). In the interior of each long cartilage the vesicular cells have insufficient nourishment, undergo rupture and disappear. As the disrupted local material is transported away a cavity forms. Mesenchyma gradually invades the cavity as it appears, thereby laying down the marrow anlage in the direction of least resistance.

The trajectorial structure of any given epiphysis can be dem-

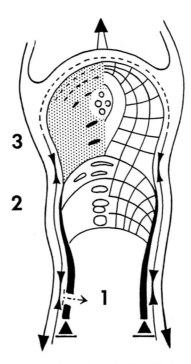

Figure 16-7. Drawing of a section through the distal end of the intermediate phalanx of a 110 mm fetus. Outlined arrow at top indicates main growth direction. Convergent arrows show growth resistance of the deep part of the periosteum. Growth resistance of the superficial part is shown by arrows directed proximally. Arrowheads represent the supporting function of the cortical bone. Trajectories of the tissue are represented by black lines. Shapes of the cells in each area are shown. *1*, diaphysis; *2*, metaphysis; *3*, epiphysis.

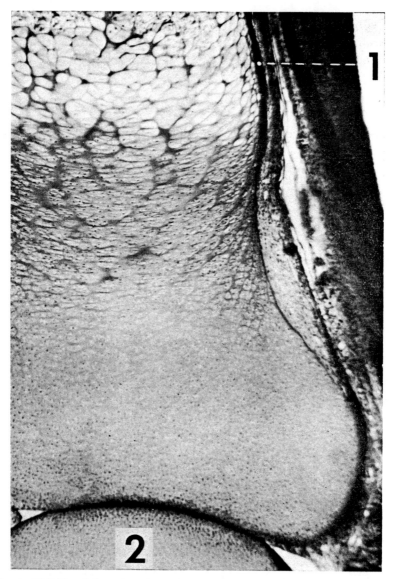

Figure 16-8. Frontal section through the distal end of the tibia of a 96 mm fetus. 100×. *1*, osseous diaphysis; *2*, head of the cartilaginous talus.

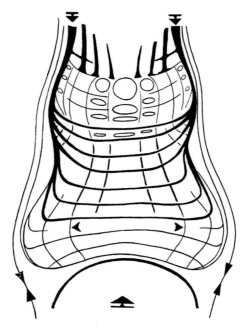

Figure 16-9. Drawing of the section shown in Figure 16-8 showing the main alignment of the cell limiting membranes (trajectorial lines) in the distal end of the tibia. Converging arrows show the restraining function of the collateral ligaments. Arrowheads indicate transverse pressure of cartilage. The upper and lower arrows with a base line indicate the longitudinal resistance of diaphyseal bone and talus, respectively.

onstrated even before it ossifies (Figs. 16-6 and 16-7). This fact demonstrates the existence of constructive developmental movements. The trajectorial arrangement which is evident supports the concept that the development of inner structure is closely related to the formation of the outer shape of the entire skeletal piece. Shape development is actually a determinant of inner structure development. Examination of the embryonic cartilaginous tibia, for example, reveals the well known trajectorial structure of the adult bone *before* ossification occurs (Figs. 16-8 and 16-9). It is difficult therefore to distinguish between so-called "work-functional-structure" (adult trajectories) and "growth-functional-structure" (embryonic trajectories).

By ignoring the size differences for a moment, one would think that the drawing in Figure 16-9 is a diagram of the spongy architecture of an adult tibia (distal end) rather that that of a fetus. By closely comparing the drawing (Fig. 16-9) with the original micrograph (Fig. 16-8) the metabolic fields of biomechanically-pressed "cushions" become evident. Fluid pressure takes place in the white zones while resistance to pull occurs in the black lines. The circular and oval structures are simple demonstrations of the column of vesicles in the cartilage. A condition for the distusion (piston) effect of the cartilage in this period is the firmness of the diaphyseal bone which has become hard and offers resistance to the growing cartilage. Arrows with base lines in Figure 16-9 show the resistance against the lengthening growth of the epiphysis. As resistance occurs, the early glenoid fossa is pressed onto the head and is consequently broadened. The structures are accordingly aligned as shown in the figure.

17

RETENSION FIELDS

ON SEVERAL OCCASIONS in preceding chapters, stretched tissue was mentioned as a special modification of inner tissue. An explanation of this finding will now be given. Stretched embryonic inner tissue is consistently observed in *retension fields*. A simplified example of the developmental movements that occur in these fields is shown in Figure 17-1. In the late developmental stages stretched inner tissue is referred to as fibrous connective tissue. A closer look will be taken of this phenomenon to try to determine what causes it. The term, retension field, signifies that an aggregation of inner tissue cells, which are initially unspecialized, grow more slowly in one particular direction than the adjacent tissue. In this manner the inner tissue cell aggregation exerts a growth resistance on the neighboring tissue. This causes a gradually increasing biomechanical counter-pull against the pulling effects of the neighboring tissue. Because "push" and "pull" never occur alone in nature, biomechanical push and pull effects should also be considered as closely related to each other. The metabolic reactions associated with such movements during human development have been scarcely investigated. However, even though this information is lacking, the following general orientation is possible.

In retension fields the morphological features of biomechanical,

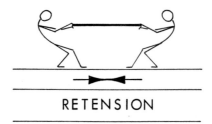

RETENSION

Figure 17-1. Simplified demonstrations of the developmental movements associated with retension fields. Two matchstick men are shown pulling on a thick rope. They tense the rope but since it does not yield, they stretch it. The stretched rope is tension-proof and exerts a greater resistance against the two matchstick men than, for example, a yielding rubber band would. Inner tissue, which is stretched by a longitudinal pull and a transverse compression, exerts a similar biomechanical resistance to growth. It acts as a restrainer (convergent arrows). Metabolic fields where mesechyma becomes stretched, thereby causing it to become a restraining apparatus, are called retension fields.

longitudinal pull in one main direction is generally associated with a simultaneous narrowing caused by transverse pressure. As an example, the mesenchymal continuations of embryonic muscle bulges will be described. Such continuations represent the anlagen of tendons, which are usually narrower than their respective muscle bulge. The mesenchymal fibers of tendon anlagen converge as they course from their respective muscle. Their convergence comes to a point where the mesenchymal fibers cross and then diverge in a fan-shaped manner into the region where the tendon inserts (Fig. 18-6, near *1*). As a general rule, all tendons are narrower than their respective muscle and have a "waist" or narrow portion where the connective tissue fibers cross (converge and diverge).

One must be cautious not to arrive at misconceptions of a mechanical consideration. It would be erroneous to believe that the tensile resistance of tendons could explain the chemistry of collagen. Likewise, it would be erroneous to say that only mechanical analyses can show this tensile resistance. Actually, many observations become clearer after both types of investigations are made separately. In addition, one would be equally mistaken to think that the metabolism and tensile resistance of stretched connective tissue are investigative subjects that contradict one another. Many observations show that there is good reason to believe that the location of chemical substances is very closely related to the biophysical origin of differentiations. For example, it is possible by means of forceps to show that stretched inner tissue and the fibrous collagenous connective tissue that appears later are greatly resistant to tensile stress. This indicates a functional relationship. Physical measurements have been made on connective tissue in later stages of development which validate this.

During the embryonic stages stretched inner tissue generally remains short. Since there have been no exceptions to this when conditions are comparable it is believed to be a rule. In light of the developmental dynamic principle which states that each part of an organism functions according to its properties at that moment, it is likely that stretched tissues act as restrainers (restraining apparatuses) even during early development. The restraining functions are united inseparably with formations that are characteristic of stretched cells. In retension fields spindle-shaped cells with slender nuclei are consistently observed within the ground substance.

One characteristic of retension is the exudation of intercellular substances from the stressed cells. This process is kinetically similar to the squeezing out of liquid contents of a porous sac when the sac is pulled longitudinally. Liquid precollagen is initially observed between cells which have become slender. After the solvent has diffused, precollagen solidifies to form the well-known micellar collagen fibers.

Postnatally, ligaments, tendons and aponeuroses always act biomechanically but in a thousand different and accurate ways. This occurs because each develops prenatally in a manner that is in harmony with the entire organism at any given moment. In adequately developed embryos collagen can always be demonstrated in locations that are compatible with the growth functions of that area. Since stretched inner tissue acts as a restrainer even during formation, it is entirely appropriate for it to restrain in the definitive condition.   This is another characteristic example of a functional development.

A characteristic feature of retension fields is that the growth resistance increases in the main direction of the inner tissue which consequently narrows.   The following is an example of this.   In Chapter 10 a frontal view of the embryonic face during the period of increased bending reveals characteristic furrows that have formed in the face area in accordance with the intense head-brain development (Fig. 10-5).   One very remarkable horizontal furrow forms between the forehead and the nose and is called the embryonic supranasal sulcus (Fig. 17-2).   Another horizontal furrow is located between the face and the cardiac bulge and is referred to as the embryonic cervical sulcus (Fig. 10-5, horizontal furrow below chin, above the head of the lower arrow).   Comparison of both regions shows similar developmental kinetics. The characteristics of a retension field are apparent and under-

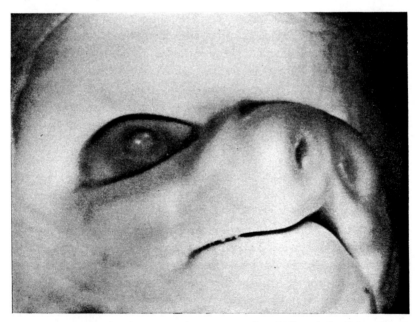

Figure 17-2. Face of a 15 mm embryo, stage 18, middle of the 7th week. A deep, horizontal supranasal sulcus appears as the forehead area protrudes and the nose tilts upwards.

standable in both of these instances, i.e. retarded growth parallel to the sulcus and narrowing of the stroma perpendicular to the direction of the sulcus. After the stroma is stretched both sulci are important in the construction of subsequent differentiations.

The stroma underneath the supranasal sulcus continues into the medial angle of the eye and into the stroma of the eyelids (Figs. 17-3 and 17-4). As it becomes narrow between the forward-bending forehead and nose, it is stretched and develops into the fibrous interorbital ligament. This ligament remains short in comparison to the expanding cerebral hemispheres. The cerebral hemispheres increase in width to a greater degree lateral to the mesencephalon (parietal part) than they do in the forehead (frontal part) where the hemispheres come into contact with each other medially. As a result of the restraining interorbital ligament, at the end of the second month, the distance between the eyes appears to be shorter in comparison to the width of the parietal part of the head. This causes the line of sight that was

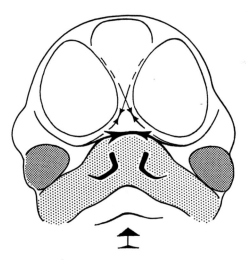

Figure 17-3. Diagram showing the restraining function of the interorbital ligament (large convergent arrows above the nose). The upwardly directed arrow below the chin represents the force from the enlarging heart. Two sets of small converging arrows show the restraining function of the brain capsule (dura mater anlage). Compare with Figure 17-4.

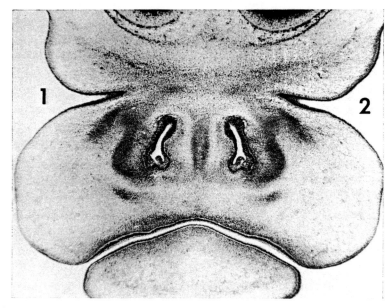

Figure 17-4. Frontal section through the face of a 17 mm (approximately) embryo, stage 19, end of the 7th week. 37×. Section is located in front of the eyes in the region of the supranasal sulcus. The ligamentous stroma beneath the sulcus (between *1* and *2*) is the interorbital ligament.

once directed lateralward now to be directed forward (compare Figs. 10-3 and 17-2).

During the C-shaped bending of the embryo the stroma beneath the cervical sulcus is hindered in growth. This becomes evident by the second month. The stroma in this area acts as a narrow collar on the ventral side of the developing neck and appears to impede the flow of lymph from the head. A large, mesh-like network is evident in the mesenchyma above this "strangling" collar. The network is biodynamically related to congestion. The mesenchymal cells bordering the network become aligned tangentially to the lymph that congests and expands the network. Consequently, they have an appearance that is similar to endothelial cells. The differentiation process that occurs in the congested region is generally referred to as the formation of the jugular lymph sacs (Fig. 17-6). After the lymph sacs have grown sufficiently, differentiation of the first lymph nodes begins. It was found to be a rule that *lymph congestion precedes the development of lymph nodes.* Lymph cells consistently develop and form the parenchyma of nodes in regions where lymph is sufficiently abundant. Lymph nodes become appropriate to certain regions because of the lymph congestion in those regions and function obviously to purify the lymph. The topogenetic principle of lymph node development in congested areas in front of "barriers" is another demonstration of the developmental dynamic differentiation of important biological processes occurring in metabolic fields that have a particular order (spatially ordered metabolic fields).

The nose is another structure that develops within stretched connective tissue and is related to the interorbital ligament. Comparison of Figures 17-3 and 17-5 shows the dura mater in the upper part of the head together with the falx cerebri ascending while the embryonic "ligament" system of the cervical viscera descends. The muzzle-like arrangement of the connective tissue in the face thereby becomes stretched in a craniocaudal direction between the falx above and the hyoid apparatus below. As a result of these two opposing, biodynamic forces, the nostrils align vertically and become longer and narrower. The thick epithelial lining of the nasal cavities grows more in the cranial and caudal directions. Simultaneous with this the nasal septum becomes longer and thinner and the previously broad mouth becomes small. In other words, the configuration of the face changes from a broad transversely aligned area to one that is narrow, vertically aligned and characteristically human (compare Figures 10-5 and 10-6).

Among all the restraining actions of stretched connective tissue, those of the tendons are particularly important. The relatively thick muscle bulges in the forearm region continue distally into the narrow fingers as tendon anlagen. In accordance with the increasing length (distusion function) of the cartilaginous phalanges (Fig. 17-7, uppermost arrow), the tendon anlagen naturally align as much as possible directly between the distal and proximal attachments of their respective muscle, taking the shortest route between the two points. As the developing digits flex, the tendon anlagen move away from the skeleton in a volar direc-

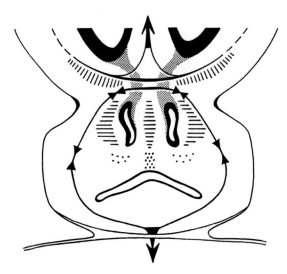

Figure 17-5. Diagram of a frontal section near the mouth of a 16 mm embryo showing the biokinetics that give rise to the vertically aligned face. The desmal skeleton (converging arrows encircling the nose and mouth) constrains the stroma in the nose-mouth area when the brain ascends (upper arrow) and the viscera descend (lower arrow). Densation fields are striped.

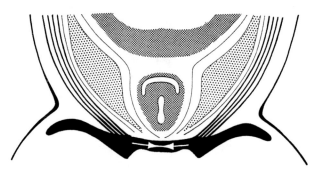

Figure 17-6. Diagram of a transverse section through the ventral neck region of a 21.5 mm embryo showing lymph congestion where the jugular lymph sacs (loosely stippled) develop. Base of skull and laryngeal area are densely stippled. Convergent arrows represent the restraining function of the stretched tissue beneath the cervical sulcus which causes the lymph congestion above it.

tion. As this occurs, they press against and stretch the adjacent volar tissue, thereby forming retinacula. This means that retinacula also differentiate in retension fields. With the increasing longitudinal growth of the phalanges, the attached retinacula spread out to form fan-shaped harnesses over the tendons.

The formation of retinacula leads to the beginning of another functional development. Because embryonic tendons are adjacent to their retinacula, longitudinal growth of the cartilaginous skele-

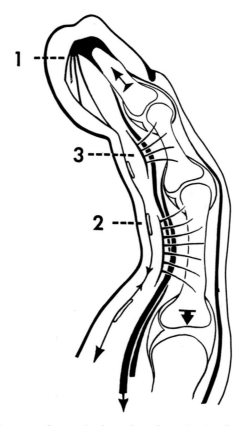

Figure 17-7. Diagram of a sagittal section through the finger of a 59 mm fetus. Divergent arrows show the distusion function of the cartilaginous pha-langes. Convergent arrows in the subcutaneous layer represent the growth resistance of blood vessels against the longitudinal growth of cartilage and cutis. *1,* connective tissue septa in subcutaneous layer; *2,* blood vessels; *3,* retinaculum.

ton in combination with the retarded growth of the tendons causes sliding movements to occur between the tendons and their retinacula. The surrounding tissue reacts to this shearing movement with the formation of clefts within which fluid accumulates. A tendon sheath differentiates as a lining of the fluid. Even the complicated arrangement of the tendon sheaths of the hand is understandable when it is viewed as being derived from local growth movements (Fig. 17-8). The dorsal flexion of the palm and the volar flexion of the fingers brings about developmental

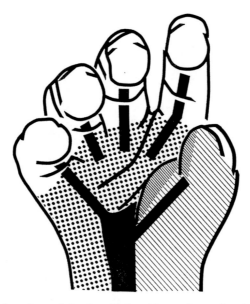

Figure 17-8. Volar view of the hand of a 46 mm fetus showing the position of the developing tendon sheaths (black zones). Tendon sheaths develop ensheathing the fluid in sliding zones which are established during dorsal flexion of the growing hand plate (proximal tendon sheaths) and volar flexion of the growing fingers (distal tendon sheaths).

movements that are positionally exact in each finger anlage. Consequently, the developmental movements are locally different giving each tendon sheath a uniquely different position, shape and structure.

With the above concept it is then relatively easy to explain the developmental dynamic principles for the structure and function of any sliding layer. This holds true for the position, time of origin and the later functions of the many fascial, bursal and joint clefts. Even though they exhibit considerable variation they are all understandable as functional differentiations with varying shearing intensities. There are no bursae, tendon sheaths or joint clefts that arise with their appropriate functions without growth functional occasions.

The retension fields in the skin (cutis) and subcutaneous (subcutis) tissue of human fetuses are of particular interest. Classical anatomists never investigated the architecture of the subcutaneous tissue perhaps because it was impossible to deduce from evolution. Eventually, its arrangement was clarified by a systematic study (cf. Blechschmidt, 1930) .[9] This study found that the shape and structure of the skin and subcutaneous tissue in all the body regions of human fetuses are specifically and uniquely human. In addition, their differentiations follow biodynamic rules. It is impossible to interpret their architecture in terms of comparative anatomy. Each area of differentiating skin represents a metabolic field with spatially ordered (directed) metabolic movements that are specific for that area. Particularly good examples to illustrate this are the skin and subcutaneous tissue on the finger tip and sole of the foot (Figs. 17-9 and 17-10) .

Examination of a sagittal section through the finger tip of a five-month fetus reveals that the skin and subcutaneous tissue occupy more space than the skeleton with nerves and blood vessels (Fig. 17-9) . The skeleton develops relatively late and occupies a position that is eccentric dorsalwards. This arrangement is in accordance with the thickness of the skin and subcutaneous layer. As was discussed earlier, the embryonic cutis is the principal forming apparatus. The epidermal part grows particularly rapidly and can be viewed as having a superficial and a deep side. The superficial part of the epidermis, called periderm, is in contact with the amniotic fluid from which it absorbs comparatively few nutrients. On the other hand, the basal part of the epidermis is in

[9]Blechschmidt, E. "Zur Anatomie des Subkutangewebes," *Z. Zellforsch*, *12*:284-293, 1930.

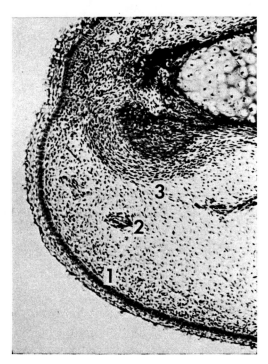

Figure 17-9. Section through the finger cushion of a 60 mm fetus. 120×. *1*, dermis; *2*, subcutaneous layer; *3*, periosteum.

contact with the underlying stroma and absorbs nutritive substances intensely. Consequently, the deeper (basal) part of the epidermis becomes thicker and more cell-crowded than the periderm (Figs. 17-9 and 19-7). The stratum intermedium lies between and connects the two sides of the epidermis.

By the third month a dermis (corium) layer is established that blends with the underlying subcutaneous layer without sharp contrast. The subcutaneous layer contains relatively few cells but much liquid intercellular substance and is therefore loose (Fig. 17-9). The subcutis is continuous by way of fibers with the fibrous layer of the skeleton. The biokinetics of this region can be interpreted from these findings.

From the biodynamic viewpoint, the epidermis becomes crowded with cells and reduced in intercellular substance because it is

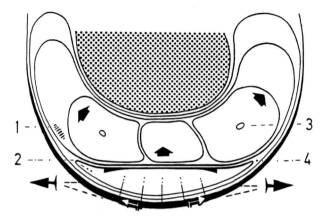

Figure 17-10. Diagram of a section through the heel pad of a 5 month fetus showing the biokinetics of the area and the typically human structure of the heel cushion. At the levels of *2* and *4* the connective tissue becomes stretched (convergent half-headed arrows) by the rapid growth of the epidermis (divergent arrows). Due to the stretching, tissue moves from the dermis towards the tuber calcanei. This movement causes the deeper part of the subcutaneous layer (subcutaneous lobules) to become compressed and to function as a cushion that protrudes laterally and medially. *1,* lamellated corpuscle; *3,* enclosed chamber with blood vessel.

able to release its katabolites in an outward direction. This results in its intense growth in relation to the deeper dermis layer. Because of the specific position of the epidermis, a metabolic gradient develops toward it from the deeper zones. The biomechanical concept of a metabolic gradient toward the body surface also explains why the young dermis is crowded with cells. It is very likely that many nutrients are located in the intercellular spaces of the subcutaneous inner tissue and flow towards the epidermis following a metabolic gradient because of the better growth conditions there. As a result of the intense supply of nutrients to the epidermis, the adjacent superficial zone of the underlying stroma is also well supplied. The cells in this zone multiply and grow rapidly causing a reduction in the size of the intercellular spaces. The space for blood vessels in the dermis thereby becomes diminished. In contrast to this, the subcutaneous zone becomes very vascular as a consequence of the metabolic gradient (Fig. 17-9, near *2*) .

Regional comparisons of various areas of the subcutaneous zone lead to the concept that the systolic pressure within the pulsating blood vessels forces fluid from the vessels into the mesenchyma tissue. This fluid causes a loosening of the subcutaneous stroma around the blood vessels. The loosened areas are the anlagen of adipose tissue lobules in the interior of which courses a blood vessel (Fig. 17-10) . The beats of the pulsating vessels stretch the stroma bordering the lobules. As a result, septa appear which divide the subcutaneous layer into chambers. The septa are tense and are tightly connected with the deeper inner tissue fibers (Fig. 17-10, connection of subcutaneous septa with the tuber calcanei) . The walls of the subcutaneous lobules become stretched in accordance with the intensity of the pulsating fluid pressure. In other words, the lobules from the moment of their inception function as cushions.

A special example of this is the subcutaneous layer on the sole of the foot which differentiates as a functional structure long before the infant stands or walks intentionally. The early functional structure is a model of the later functional structure of the adult heel cushion.

At the beginning of the second month, the ectoderm on the medial side of the fold-like anlage of the lower extremity (sole area) is reduced in area and becomes thicker as the anlage undergoes growth adduction (cf. 1973, p. 86) . Not only is the ectoderm thickened but also the underlying stroma that supplies it. Even in embryos the arteries in the subcutis become strong. As surface growth of the embryonic sole cutis is hindered, it appears to be compressed proximodistally. As surface growth is hindered, the stroma thickens and becomes crowded with cells and reduced in intercellular substance. This zone thereby becomes the especially well-developed dermis. Because of the thickened ectoderm the requirements for nutrients increase, the underlying blood vessels enlarge and become more numerous. The increased vascularity of the sole area causes it to have an intense red color.

As a result of the rapid growth of the superficial layer of the fetal skin the basal part of the dermis which is relatively retarded in growth, becomes stretched and flattened (Fig. 17-10, convergent arrows in fibrous layer). During this process the stretched part of the dermis (oldest zone) displaces from the curved overlying epidermis and approaches the underlying tuber calcanei. As this movement occurs, the subcutaneous layer of the heel between the fibrous layer and the calcaneus is compressed and functions biomechanically as a cushion (Fig. 17-10). This takes place long before any pressure from walking is exerted on the heel. As the fibrous layer moves away from the epidermis the intervening stroma becomes loosened. This stromal loosening allows peripheral sweat glands to grow down into the layer of the heel cushion which is the youngest layer (*see* Chapter 19).

18

DILATION FIELDS

THE PRINCIPLES which precartilage, cartilage, tendons and ligaments follow during their origin were given in the preceding chapters. The question of whether or not there are principles followed during the origin of muscle will be answered in this chapter. Developing cells and cell aggregations differ more and more from each other. As a result of this and from what has been said earlier, it can be concluded that the developmental movements of cells (determined from observations on staged series), as well as their developmental dynamics, are different. Developing muscles differ from one location to another but one should expect to find principles which all muscles follow during their origin.

The fields in which musculature arises are defined in very exact terms and are spatially and kinetically highly organized. Blechschmidt has named them *dilation fields* (Fig. 18-1). The term "dilation" but not "dilatation" is intentionally used in order to avoid confusion with the latter word whose meaning has only a mechanical connotation. The principal of muscle origin in dilation fields is valid for the anlage of skeletal, cardiac and smooth muscle fibers and fiber systems. Here the unity of the fiber systems is demonstrable in spite of the variety of individual characteristics. When the place of origin of musculature is investigated, it be-

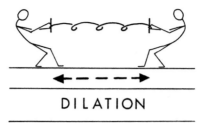

DILATION

Figure 18-1. Simplified demonstration of the developmental movements associated with dilation fields. Two matchstick men are shown pulling apart an easily extensible spiral spring. As they pull on the spring it gives way to the pull with little resistance and becomes slenderer. Embryonic tissue such as mesenchyma becomes elongated and slendered by growth pull in a particular direction (divergent arrows with interrupted stems). Inner tissue which is stretched by a longitudinal pull *without* transverse compression is a dilation field.

comes evident that the shape of the musculature is closely related to its position and its structure is closely related to its shape.

Some examples will now be given to demonstrate some characteristics that are common to all developing muscles. A prime example is the differentiation of the X-shaped heart anlage on the dorsal wall of the pleuropericardial (thoracic) part of the early embryonic coelom (Chapter 5). The heart anlage becomes filled with, and distended by blood that has a high osmotic pressure. During the period of early development the cardiac wall is very likely less pressed by the coelomic fluid on its outside than by the blood on its inside, since blood has a higher osmolarity than coelomic fluid. As a result, the heart anlage is stimulated to dilate. In fact, a distinct growth dilation is evident in embryos over 3 mm. For instance, in stage 11 (Fig. 18-2) the cardiac muscle anlagen immediately beneath the epicardium can regularly be observed to be dilated precisely circular to the longitudinal axis of the cardiac tube, i.e. parallel to the drawn hatched lines. As the cardiac tube lengthens and widens, the anlagen of the cardiac muscle cells become larger and, like all muscle cells, more slender.

The explanation for this is as follows: The cardiac tube is the only embryonic blood capillary which, because of its position in

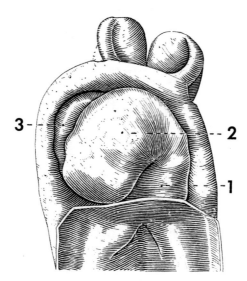

Figure 18-2. Ventral view of the early heart of a 3.1 mm embryo, stage 11, 13 somites, approximately 23 days (Blechschmidt embryo). The heart at this period of development is an intensely growing folded tube suspended from the dorsal wall of the pleuropericardial cavity. *1*, inflow path; *2*, connecting piece; *3*, outflow path (for positional relationships *see* Blechschmidt, 1973, p. 8).

the thoracic part of the coelomic cavity, has the space to expand and the occasion to dilate early and quickly between the osmotic pressure in the interior of the cardiac tube and the pressure outside in the coelomic fluid. In the illustrated stage the cardiac muscle fibers have become very spindle-shaped during systole. They respond to the dilation, gradually reacting in vivo by contracting. It has been known for some time that dilations and contractions alternate during early development. During diastole fluid accumulates between the embryonic endothelium (endocardium) and the myoepicardium. During systole, when the epithelial endocardium is less dilated and consequently is probably less permeable, not all of the fluid returns to the lumen of the vessel. As a result, the cells within the cardiac wall are able to shift against each other.

In the fourth week the early cardiac tube, which is never quite symmetrical, progressively dilates. This, in turn, increases the dilation resistance of the circular musculature. Growth of the cardiac tube in its given cavity conforms to the dilation resistance of the circular musculature. The cardiac tube lengthens and, because it is fixed at each end to the walls of the "thoracic" cavity, bends into an omega shape. The connecting piece is especially mobile and bends at first convexly to the left but later convexly ventralward and then to the right (Fig. 18-2). Before the end of the first month the connecting piece, dilating by growth, becomes so large in comparison to the inflow and outflow paths that it aligns from left to right, i.e. in the main dimension of the early coelom. The growth dilation of the left and right ventricles begins in this manner. At this stage the connecting piece forms as a loop that attaches to the anlage of the diaphragm (septum transversum). As a result of this differentiation, the early heart at the stage illustrated no longer represents a tube that is nearly circular on transverse section but becomes a tortuous tube with increasingly distinct flattenings (1973, p. 46).

Concurrently, the somites (Chapter 6) also exhibit the general biodynamic principle of growth dilation in the region of myotome formation. The following has been discovered from making regional comparisons. The cranial and caudal edges of the dermatome portion of the somites grow very rapidly in the direction of least resistance, i.e. cranially and caudally (Figs. 18-3 to 18-5). This occurs in accordance with lengthening of the whole embryo. Consistent with this growth, the cells underneath the dermatomes become aligned in a craniocaudal manner that corresponds to the increasing distance between the dorsal intersegmental (metameric) veins (Fig. 18-3). During this process, new cells from the multiplying dermatome cells lie on the developing myotome thereby forming a vortex as shown in Figures 18-4 and 18-5. It is in this region that the first dorsal musculature appears underneath the dermatome and parallel to the longitudinal axis of the growing neural tube. The young muscle cells become slender in the dilation field and, at the same time, longitudinally-arranged fibrils develop in their interior. Transverse striations are initially ill-defined.

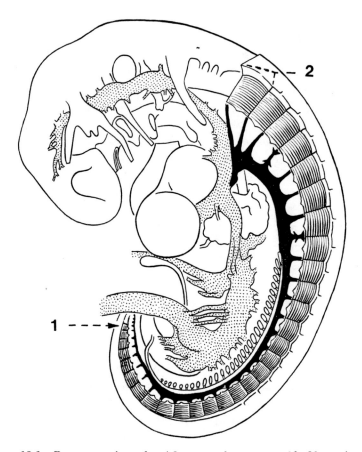

Figure 18-3. Reconstruction of a 4.2 mm embryo, stage 13, 20 somites, approximately 28 days. As the embryo progressively bends and lengthens the distances between the metameric veins enlarge particularly peripherally. Convergent arrows indicate the restraining function of the veins. *1,* most caudal myotome; *2,* most cranial myotome.

After the first month characteristic rows of nuclei become distinct (Fig. 18-5, middle portion) as a result of the lengthening of the muscle cells. Initially, the nuclei are not flat and do not yet lie at the periphery of the cell. Because of this arrangement, early striated muscle cells are similar to smooth muscle cells. As the dermatome cells become aligned perpendicular to the basement

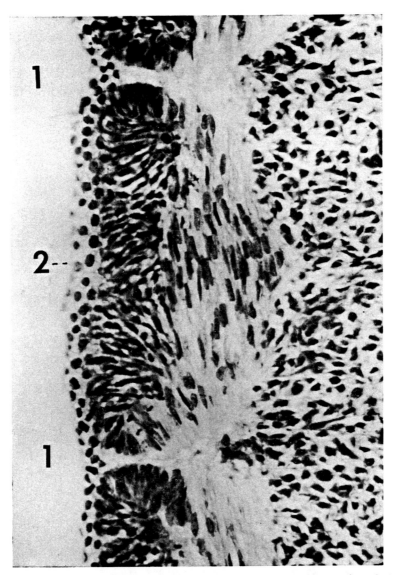

Figure 18-4. A longitudinal section through a differentiating somite of the upper back region of the same 4.2 mm embryo shown in Figure 18-3. 440×. The ectoderm is on the left margin. The dark cell-crowded dermatome beneath the ectoderm is obliquely cut. Medial to the dermatome (on the right) is the myotome that is rich in intercellular substance and therefore stains light. Height of this particular myotome is 0.2 mm. *1*, segmentation septa; *2*, intrasegmental zone.

membrane of the ectoderm (Figs. 18-4 and 18-5), the tapering myotomes and myotome cells are positioned perpendicular to the segmentation septa. The alignment of the cells in the dermatomes should be considered as a sign of active surface growth resulting in the passive alignment of the myotome cells.

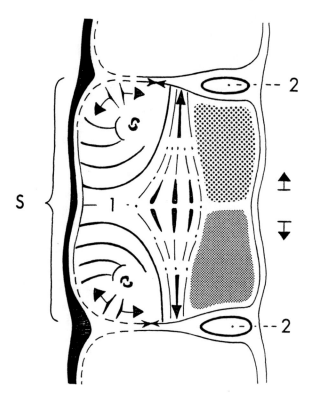

Figure 18-5. Diagram of the same section through a differentiating somite shown in Figure 18-4 indicating the developmental kinetics. Growth dilation of the myotome is shown by the long diverging arrows in the middle. The somite bulge of the ectoderm (S) is on the left border. The growth of the spinal cord is represented by the divergent arrows with base lines on the right. Main growth zone of the dermatome is indicated by two sets of divergent arrows with base lines near the ectoderm. Converging arrows at the periphery of the somite show the retension of the segmentation septa. Area of the developing spinal nerve is indicated with large coarse stippling; area of the developing skeleton (sclerotome) is shown with fine dense stippling. *1*, site of an intrasegmental gap; *2*, segmentation septa with veins.

In each dilation field the spatial opportunity and the developmental dynamic occasion are generally present for the development of the bulged part of the slender muscle cells as well as of the thin tendons. Normal muscle development is never observed as an isolated process of self-differentiation. It can always be demonstrated from regional comparisons that the bulging shape of the muscle cells and the muscle themselves are characteristic of the growth processes in dilation fields. In other words, dilation fields are characterized not only by the longitudinal dilation of the immature cells but also, to a lesser extent, by dilation in a direction that is transverse to the longitudinal one. As the longitudinal dilation increases, the muscle cells become slender but remain bulgy. The myotomes do not differ in this feature from any later skeletal musculature.

Postnatally, the slendering of muscles increases over many years corresponding to the growth of surrounding structures. This occurs in the entire muscle as well as in each muscle fiber. An important rule is as valid here as it is for other complicated differentiations, i.e. there is a similarity of the structures developing at different orders of magnitude. In this sense, the following are comparable: Muscles and muscle fibers; tendons and tendon fibers; glands and gland lobes; primary gut loops and secondary gut loops; kidneys and renal lobes; long bones and osteones. The component of each pair is similar to the other in its form but in a different order of magnitude.

Muscle anlagen in narrowed zones have no opportunity to bulge but, in contrast, narrow transversely to their main dilation direction. In these regions they develop tendons. Dilation in conjunction with transverse compression is characteristic of the differentiations described in a retension field (Chapter 17). Transverse compression is always found in the metabolic fields of the embryonic tendon anlagen (at the tips of the myotomes). This is illustrated in Figure 18-6, near *1*. In this region, the water content of the intercellular substance is reduced and subsequently the intercellular substance is consolidated. Histologically, the region becomes progressively more stainable. With regard to the early tips of the myotomes where tendons form, possibly the solvent of precollagen which exudes from the tips of the muscle cells diffuses into the neighboring blood vessels. Perhaps in this manner the myotome cells are drawn toward the segmentation septa. When tissue locally has become tendinous it cannot be dilated biomechanically like the bulges of muscles. Like all stretched tissue, embryonic tendons also show restraining functions. Restraining functions with a relatively low tensile state in comparison to the growing muscle bulges are characteristic of such structures as the tendons of the long flexors and extensors of the fingers, aponeuroses and intermuscular septa. There are numerous examples of

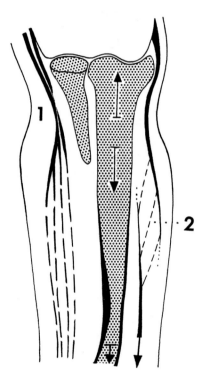

Figure 18-6. Drawing of a frontal section through elbow and proximal forearm areas of a 41 mm fetus, 3rd month. Dilation fields where skeletal muscle develop are shown. Diverging arrows with base line represent the longitudinal (distusion) growth of the cartilaginous ulna. Simple arrow indicates the growth pull of a tendon. *1,* crossing tendon fibers at the end of a muscle bulge; *2,* obliquely arranged muscle fibers near tendons (dilation field).

this principle but a well-known one is the aponeurosis of the trapezius muscle between the skin and the deeper dorsal muscles.

With regard to the normal development of skeletal musculature, embryonic cartilage plays a most important role. The distusion function of embryonic cartilage is essential to the growth dilation of muscles and for the stretching of tendons (Figs. 18-6 to 18-8). All of the dilation fields of skeletal muscles develop

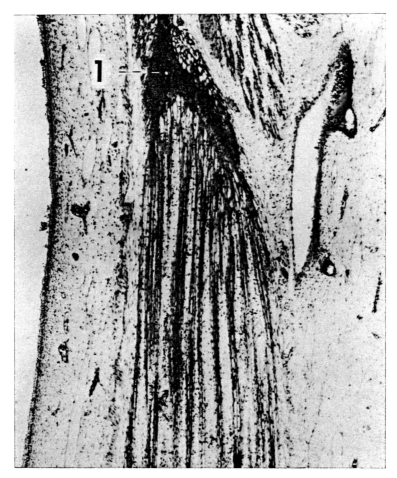

Figure 18-7. Longitudinal section through skeletal muscle of a 50 mm fetus. 55×. *1*, site where a tendon is forming as a "thimble" on the tapering end of a muscle bulge (*see* Figure 18-6).

kinetically in accordance with the swelling growth of cartilage on which the distusion function of the latter depends. On the basis if this swelling growth, the neighboring tissue that is at first undifferentiated becomes functioning musculature by means of growth dilation. If the developmental movements of the cartilaginous skeleton are known, the origin and development of the function of each muscle can be deduced. This means that initially, when compared with embryonic cartilage, all muscles have passive forming functions before they are able to actively contract. Many examples of this can be given. No muscle can shorten by means of contraction if it has not first become sufficiently long. In order to become long and slender, the muscle regularly needs space. In other words, each muscle needs the circumstances that are stimuli for its development of functions. Organs always differentiate by subdivision of the whole and never by the composition of isolated parts.

If one compares the distances of the so-called origins and insertions of the muscles in dilation fields one finds that the distances

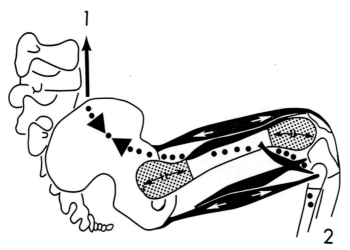

Figure 18-8. Hip and lower extremity regions of a 50 mm fetus showing distusion (diverging arrows with base lines in cartilaginous portion of femur) and dilation (diverging simple arrows in extensor and flexor muscles) fields. Dotted line between *1* and *2* represents the restraining function (convergent arrow heads) of the femoral vessels (*see* Figure 12-16).

increase in accordance with cartilage growth, i.e. muscle bulges that have different locations usually become slender at a variable rate. Without the fast dilation movement, muscles probably would not obtain their normal innervation (Chapter 9). As a rule, when growing muscle cells lengthen quickly, they obtain a rich innervation. As a result they are able to contract quickly. In the later stages of development such muscles are capable of quick, voluntary movements.

Dilation fields are also observed in the intestinal tract. Such fields indicate particularly the localization and early development of functions of the smooth musculature. A characteristic example is the musculature of the gut. As a result of growth of the endoderm, a metabolic gradient is established which is regularly followed by vascularization of the intestinal wall near the endoderm. The pressure in the pulsating blood vessels appears to support the expansion effort of the endoderm as the gut lumen widens. The circular arrangement of the stromal cells shows the growth pressure of the inner layer of the gut and demonstrates that the motor for the forming work of the embryonic intestinal tube resides in the epithelium. Because of the forming function of the epithelium the mesenchymal cells differentiate into circularly arranged musculature. In regard to the difference between the forming function of skeletal and smooth musculature, the latter could be named epithelial musculature because of its topokinetic relationship to the epithelium. The cells of the smooth musculature of the intestine are dilated in spatially exact positions by the strong surface growth of the endodermal epithelium (Fig. 18-9).

Based on what is now known, the following concept is being considered as a kinetic principle of differentiation. A dilation field occurs around the expanding system of endoderm together with its neighboring vascularized stroma. In such a field the early muscle cells have a growth direction that is mainly circular. After this field has enlarged sufficiently, that is, the entire tissue aggregation has grown, the circularly arranged cells exert an increasing growth resistance on the endoderm. As a result of the increasing growth resistance (arranged circularly) the gut then grows more in length with the stroma, between the serosal epithelium and the

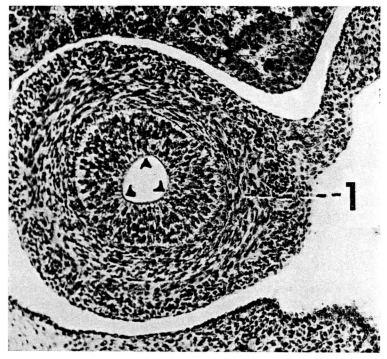

Figure 18-9. Transverse section through the small intestine of an 18.5 mm embryo, stage 20, 8th week. 150×. Arrowheads show the widening of the gut lumen by growth of its epithelial lining. A dilation field *(1)* is established adjacent to the vascular zone peripheral to the expanding endoderm giving origin to the circular layer of smooth muscle.

circular musculature, developing into the longitudinal musculature.

The gut is another example of how exact the developmental kinetic relationships are between position, shape and structure. The lumen in the more cranial part of the gut is filled by the secretions of the great intestinal glands (liver and pancreas). Because of the filling this portion of the gut widens before the more caudal portion. Initially, the proximal segment of the small intestine is usually wide and the caudal segment is narrow. The embryonic colon is particularly narrow. Only later do the proportions change. In the beginning of the second month, i.e. in the beginning of the specific embryonic period the narrow colon exhibits a very small lumen that has three angles on transverse sections (Fig. 18-10). Studies on the developmental movements of the embryonic colon show that the blood vessels that form on the side of the mesentery grow into the intestinal wall and therefore hinder surface growth of the mesenteric portion of the endoderm by their retarded growth in accordance with the rule presented in Chapter 8. Because of this, the endoderm on the mesenteric side of the embryonic colon thickens and protrudes into the intestinal lumen (Fig. 18-10, central outlined arrow). In contrast, the laterally adjacent (paramesenteric) epithelium (near *2*) is pushed outwards as the anlage of a haustrum. In the region where surface growth of the endoderm is hindered the stroma becomes

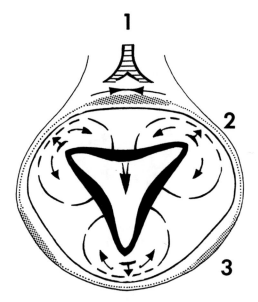

Figure 18-10. Transverse section through the colon of a 50 mm fetus showing the developmental kinetics that give rise to haustra and taeniae coli. Arrows with a base line represent main growth pressure of the lining epithelium (solid black zone) and diverging arrows indicate alignment of the stroma. Converging arrows at the attachment of the mesocolon (*1*) represent the restraining function of the branching blood vessels here. Large outlined arrow shows growth direction of the protruding epithelium on the mesenteric side. *2*, location of haustrum; *3*, site of taenia coli.

aligned perpendicular to the basement membrane (ends of the broken lines in Fig. 18-10). In the paramesenteric zone, where the epithelium is less hindered in surface growth, the adjacent layer of tissue is aligned more circularly but is free of muscle cells. Only peripherally does a satisfactorily strong dilation field occur where the well-known circular musculature develops. Externally, the longitudinal musculature develops between three rows of haustra forming the taeniae coli (stippled zones near *3* in Fig. 18-10). In this manner, the wall of the colon receives a specific differentiation that is different from that of the small intestine. Such observations force one to conceive of metabolic fields with spatially ordered metabolic movements.

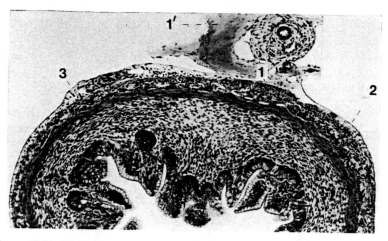

Figure 18-11. Transverse section through the colon of an 80 mm fetus showing the early temporary formation of villi. 350×. *1,* taenia coli; *1',* mesentery; *2* and *3,* haustra.

The wide small intestine shows other features of differentiation which are also understandable in kinetic terms. Its endoderm quickly increases in surface area and forms intestinal glands (crypts) and villi earlier than in the colon (Fig. 18-11). The cell nuclei of the crypts and villi have specific positions. The crypts, being in close contact with the stroma, exhibit intense cell multiplication followed by cell growth. Intense surface enlargement occurs in the region of the crypts that is related to the cell multiplication. As the surface enlarges in these areas, the adjacent

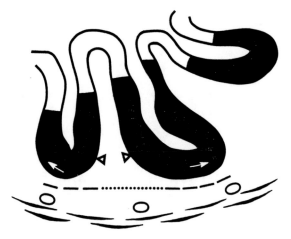

Figure 18-12. Diagram of a transverse section through the small intestine of a 50 mm fetus showing the developmental kinetics that give rise to the muscularis mucosae as a result of growth of the epithelium (diverging white arrows). The growing crypts move apart from each other (arrowheads). Dotted line shows the position of the dilation field (muscularis mucosae).

epithelium of the villi is pushed into the intestinal lumen and detaches from its underlying tissue. Here, many villi are established in a short time. The lightly stained areas in the tips of the villi are a sign that these areas contain much water. This brings one to the conclusion that in the region of the villi metabolic movements are from the lumen into the wall, whereas in the region of the crypts, the movements occur with extensive assimilation of nourishment from the stroma and the delivery of cell products into the intestinal lumen. If this is true, it would mean that spatially ordered metabolic movements are a predevelopment of glandular function. As the growing glands move apart from each other and enlarge the surrounding tissue, the region between the glands becomes dilated, thereby forming the muscularis mucosae (Figs. 18-11 and 18-12).

19

PARATHELIAL LOOSENING FIELDS

NOT ONLY DENSATION fields but also *loosening fields* occur among tissue differentiations. Loosening fields are characterized by congestion of the intercellular substance in the inner tissue into which katabolites of the cells are released. As the volume of the katabolites increases the volume of the intercellular substance enlarges and the vesicles fuse together (Fig. 19-1). At early stages of development these loosening areas within the mesoderm are precursors of arising pathways preparing for blood vessel formation (Chapter 8).

Among loosening zones a special group occurs which are called *parathelial* (paraepithelial) *suction fields*. The developmental kinetics of such fields are illustrated in Figure 19-2. Differentiations occurring in these fields are typical for glands. A feature

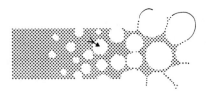

LOOSENING FIELD

Figure 19-1. Diagram of a loosening field which is caused by congestion of liquid intercellular substances in the inner tissue.

common to the beginning of both exocrine and endocrine glands is early loosening of the stroma at their point of origin. The epithelial anlage of the gland grows into the loosened stroma. The manner of development of labial glands will be used as an example.

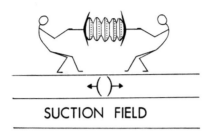

SUCTION FIELD

Figure 19-2. Simplified demonstration of the developmental movements associated with suction fields. Two matchstick men pull apart a bellows. As they pull a lower pressure arises in the bellows. Embryonic inner tissue which is stressed in such a manner becomes loosened (divergent arrows). Inner tissue which is loosened by being stretched out in three dimensions is referred to as a suction field.

The distusion growth of the cartilaginous nasal capsule and lower jaw causes the skeleton supporting the mouth to open. Thereby, the dorsoventral dimension of the embryonic face increases as a result of the enlargement and lengthening of the cartilages and the distance between the gingivae of the upper and lower jaws increases. As a result of this, the stroma in the interior of the embryonic upper and lower lips dilates in a circular direction around the mouth opening, thereby forming the orbicularis oris muscle. As is usual in dilation fields, growth in this area is retarded relative to the extending structures. This is evident from the fact that the lips at this time of development roll inward (Fig. 19-3, curved outlined arrows). The soft parts of the mouth thereby approach each other closing the mouth opening. In biophysical terms the orbicularis oris muscle functioning as a dilation resistance assists in the formation of the lips even at the time of their development, not only during the postnatal period.

As a result of the inward rolling of the lips, surface growth of

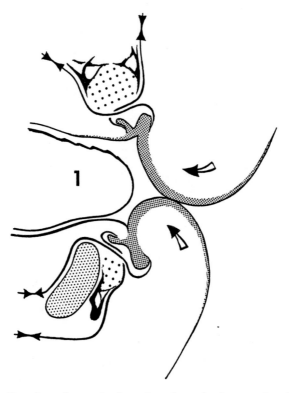

Figure 19-3. Drawing of a sagittal section through the mouth of a 29 mm embryo, stage 23, end of second month showing some of the developmental kinetics of this area. Inrolling movements of the lips (curved outlined arrows) cause immediately the formation of the thickened epithelial jaw ledges (laminae) as areas hindered in growth. Convergent arrows represent the restraining function of the skeletal connective tissue. Labial epithelium is finely stippled, areas of arising osseous alveoli are largely stippled. Intermediate stipple shows area of Meckel's cartilage. *1*, tongue.

the overlying mucosal epithelium is hindered (convergent arrows in Fig. 19-4). Growth is mainly hindered in the transitional region of the lips where they join the floor or roof of the embryonic mouth. In these two transitional regions there appear solid epithelial thickenings called jaw ledges (labiodental laminae). Near the end of the second month and the beginning of the third month the ledges broaden. Consequently, they appear to be spread out when observed in sagittal sections (Fig. 19-3) . The two parts of the spread ledge are referred to as the labial (vestibular) ledge and the dental ledge when considered as isolated parts.

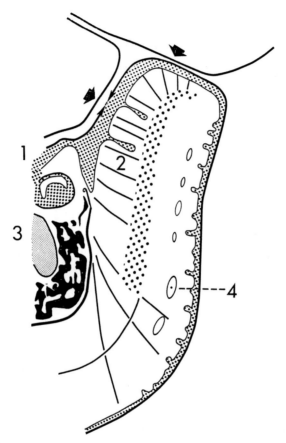

Figure 19-4. Drawing of a sagittal section through the lower lip of an 80 mm fetus showing the appearance of labial glands in parathelial suction fields. Black arrows indicate the growth resistance of the neighboring organs, i.e. tongue and upper lip. Convergent arrows indicate retarded growth and consequent restraining function of the superficial mucosa epithelium. Growth dilation of the orbicularis oris muscle (coarse stipple) increases as a result of the pressure of the fluid squeezed from the mucosal epithelium. As the growth dilation increases the stroma deep to the mucosa thickens forming a suction field. The epithelium forms the labial glands in the suction field by its deep surface growth. *1*, general dental ledge; *2*, zone of loosened stroma; *3*, Meckel's cartilage with outer zone of mandibular bone; *4*, blood vessel.

Growth and differentiation of the two subdivisions are required for normal development of the teeth (cf. 1961).

When the mucosal epithelium of the embryonic lips is sufficiently thick its superficial and deep portions begin to differ. Superficially, the epithelium adjacent to the fluid of the oral cavity grows slowly because its supply of nutritive substances is very limited. On the other hand, the deep portion adjacent to the nutritive stroma enlarges rapidly. Water accumulates in the stroma which indicates that the decomposition (katabolism) products of metabolism (mainly water) are not released to the outside but toward the inside.

Blood vessels of the skin also play a role in these differentiation processes. It is evident that blood vessels form a very strong network which probably is widened by each systole. The authors have never observed a living embryo that does not show pulsatoric deformations. Because of this phenomenon most developmental movements probably occur in an undulating manner rather than rectilinearly.

During the inrolling of the lips the stromal cells regularly align perpendicular to the basement membrane. Intercellular substance accumulates in the interstices of the cells. The stroma obtains a loose appearance in the area where the intercellular substance accumulates (Fig. 19-4, white areas in layer 2). Figure 19-5 shows how the stratum basale (black layer) of the epithelium adapts to the loosening by increased surface growth along the stroma. This epithelium forms the anlagen of club-shaped glands in the direction of least resistance. The anlagen grow into the cell interstices of the stroma as a result of the extensive assimilation that takes place at their club-shaped ends. Here the cells diverge as a broad cone towards the stroma. In a way, they grow by "sucking" into the loosened stroma. Once a gland arises the stratum basale is relieved of the cell crowding. Consequently, the origin of each gland prevents the development of another gland in its immediate vicinity.

A study of the growth of labial glands reveals the following developmental kinetic principle. Wedge epithelium with pyramid-shaped cells occurs in the round tip of the early gland where it lies

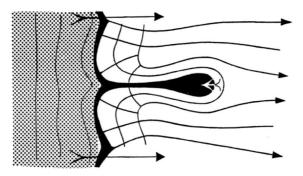

Figure 19-5. Enlarged drawing of a labial gland anlage from Figure 19-4 showing that its growth direction is orthogonal (long arrows) to its matrix (mucosa membrane). Black-tailed arrows represent the flow of liquid from the epithelium into the adjacent stroma. White-tailed arrow depicts the absorption of nutritive substance from the stroma by the glandular tip. The mucosal epithelium is stippled with its stratum basale in solid black. The parathelial suction field is white.

adjacent to the stroma. The cell limits of wedge epithelium are aligned nearly radial to the center of the glandular tip. On the other hand, where the tip joins the rest of the epithelium, there occurs prismatic wedge epithelium as is characteristic for all tube-shaped cell aggregations (Fig. 5-4). The cell nuclei in the glandular tip migrate to the broader side of the cell near the stroma where assimilation takes place. There they become spherical. Numerous mitoses occur in this location and surface growth becomes intense. Consequently, local growth rate of the epithelium forming the tip of the labial glands is more intense than that of the excretory duct with which it is continuous.

As surface growth of the glandular tip increases a lumen appears in its interior. As a result of polarization of the epithelium a dissimilation side of the tip develops where fluid is released by the epithelium. Simultaneous with this the summit of the gland anlage recedes towards the lumen causing the tip to subdivide (Fig. 19-6). Adenomeres (cells in the blind terminal portions of a developing gland) form because of these metabolic movements that are characteristic of polarized limiting tissues. As a result of their further surface growth and subsequent dichotomic subdivision, the glandular tree begins to develop. The general validity of developmental dynamic differentiations is indicated by the similarity of such gland anlagen to the ureteric tree, the growing bronchial tree and other similarly branched formations.

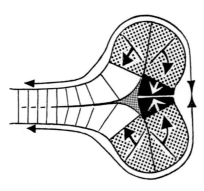

Figure 19-6. Drawing of the growing acinus of a labial gland showing the biokinetics of adenomere formation. Surface growth of the epithelium against an outer resistance (convergent arrows) causes the development of adenomeres (gland cells). Arrows with a base line indicate the direction of growth. Finely stippled area is the lumen. Largely stippled cells undergo accelerated growth whereas solid black cells undergo reduced growth.

If a glandular excretory duct ruptures as a result of the positional relationship between the gland and the descending viscera, then the gland anlage becomes ductless and consequently an endocrine gland. The development of several such endocrine glands was explained in Chapter 8. The origin of the suprarenal gland is a special situation that should be mentioned here in order to show that even very complex differentiations are subordinate to simple rules. During the origin of the suprarenal gland, cells of the limiting tissue (serosa) grow into the loose environment along with the ganglion cells that form the medulla. This growth occurs in the direction of least resistance, that is, subserosal (parathelial). When the liver expands by growth, this parathelial field develops in the area of transition of the serosa on the liver to that on the dorsal body wall.

From the above examples it should be evident that glands

originate in a regular manner. All glands thus far investigated appear in a parathelial field that is a loosely arranged suction zone next to epithelia (Fig. 19-2). Their appearance is part of the total growth process of the embryo. There is nothing that suggests that any epithelial appendage can find its place or origin independently, without an external, localized occasion that has specific spatial dimensions.

At this time it might be well to discuss some of the more specific differentiations of the skin appendages. Because the skin is an outer organ it is of particular importance in the differentiation process since differentiation has been shown again and again to occur from the outside inwards. It may be recalled that in the early entocyst (embryonic) disc, the appearance of the embryo was initially a result of ectodermal formations. During the entire subsequent period of development the skin and its precursors have been recognized again and again as the primary forming apparatus.

During the increasing growth of the embryo the skin exhibits more and more local differences as its cells increase in number and the volume of the stroma enlarges. The spatial circumstances of even the skin are important for its normal differentiation processes. In a typical stage (Fig. 19-7) the epidermis, e.g. of the finger cushion, has three layers: (1) a thin, membrane-like cell layer superficially in contact with the amniotic fluid, called the *periderm,* which has a low mitotic rate; (2) a thick, deep layer, the *stratum basale,* where assimilation occurs on its deep side and there is intense multiplication and resultant growth of the cells; and (3) a specific connecting layer between these two limiting layers called the *stratum intermedium* (light zone in Figs. 19-7 and 19-8).

The intense surface growth of the stratum basale produces peaks and valleys causing the layer to undulate. As a result of this the corium of the fetus which is always crowded with cells forms more complicated structures than previously. The wedge epithelium of the peaks next to the stroma forms crest-like folds containing large cells and numerous mitoses. The mitoses are absent in the epithelial valleys between the crests. The folds have an

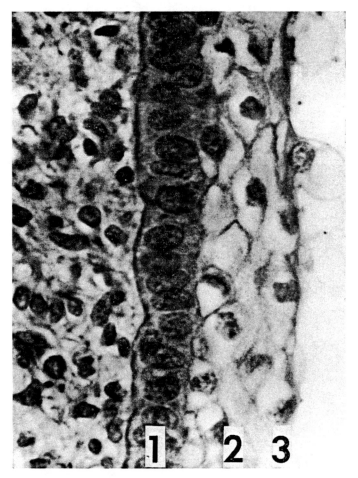

Figure 19-7. Sagittal section through the finger cushion of a 59 mm fetus. 100×. *1*, stratum basale; *2*, stratum intermedium; *3*, periderm.

effect even on the outer surface (Fig. 19-9). They are the anlagen of the papillary system of ridges in the fingers and show individual variations.

In order to avoid any misunderstanding with regard to the importance of the genes, the following example is given. In the manufacturing industry microtome knives with the thinnest edges are produced from raw material which was, for example, collected at one time from mine **X** and at another time from mine **Y**. After long, technical treatment of the material it becomes evident that the knives made from the material from one mine are of better quality than those made from the material from the other mine. Does this mean that the material contains an imprint to produce a knife of a particular quality? Not at all! Features of anlage materials often become important late in the differentiation pro-

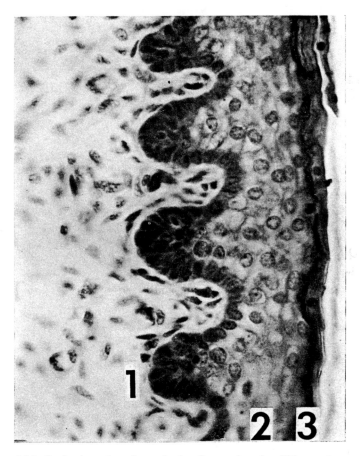

Figure 19-8. Sagittal section through the finger tip of a 110 mm human fetus. 630×. The stratum basale (*1*) has changed into wedge epithelium with many mitotic figures. This is the growth area from which sweat glands arise. *2* and *3* as in Figure 19-7.

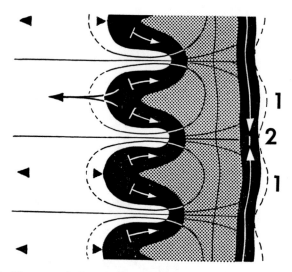

Figure 19-9. Diagram of the section in Figure 19-8 showing the biokinetics of sweat gland formation. The accumulation of liquid in the parathelial fields is indicated by broken-lined arcades. The liquid moves from the stratum basale (tailed arrow). The pressure of the intercellular liquid is indicated by arrowheads. White arrows with a base line show the direction of growth in the stratum basale. Growth direction of the sweat glands is perpendicular to their matrix. The resistance of the outer epithelial stratum (convergent white arrows) causes the formation of papillary ledges or ridges (*1*) and furrows (*2*).

cess. A similar situation is true for the role that genes play in the differentiation process.

The fluid metabolic products of the epithelial cells (Fig. 19-9, tailed arrow) collect near the folds of the papillary system which are directed basalward with their convexity toward the stroma. In these parathelial fields loosened by fluid the basal cell layer gives rise to sweat glands perpendicular (90° angle) to the epidermis. What is true for "soft" epithelial appendages is also valid with modifications for "hard" epithelial appendages such as hairs. Contrary to sweat glands, hair anlagen are usually inclined against the epithelial layer forming an angle of about 45°. This inclination is understandable only when one becomes aware of positional relationships. In other words, one must first know the con-

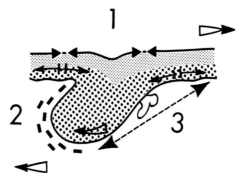

Figure 19-10. Diagram of a section through the developing hair germ (follicle) from an 80 mm fetus showing the developmental movements of this formation. Outlined arrows at the top and bottom show the opposite movements of the epithelium and the underlying stroma. This causes the main growth direction of the hair germ to be inclined to its matrix (curved outlined arrow). Convergent arrows indicate the retarded growth of the outer epithelial stratum. Divergent arrows with base lines show the rapid surface growth of the stratum basale (fine stipple). *1*, depression of the periderm; *2*, retension field; *3*, dilation field where the arrector pili muscle arises.

nections the hair anlagen have with the entire developing organism considered as a whole. Investigations performed with the developmental kinetic points of view show the following relationships. In most areas of the body of the growing fetus, the epidermis grows toward the apex of the trunk, that is, caudalward in the direction of least resistance.[10] In so doing it glides on the underlying layer of tissue. As a result of this movement the protrusions of the stratum basale begin to tilt in relation to the stratum superficiale as the cells multiply and grow. Short rolling movements of the basal protrusions occur (Fig. 19-10, large curved arrow). Because of these movements the epithelial hair anlagen usually grow into the stroma as oblique protrusions of the epidermis. As a result of these developmental movements, the stroma in each acute angle between the epidermis and the hair anlage become compressed but loosen in the obtuse angle on the other

[10]Blechschmidt, E. "Die konstruktive Entwicklung des kraniokaudalen Haarstrichs," *Anat. Anz 83,* 1937.

longer side of the anlage (Fig. 19-10, compressed at *2* and loosened at *3*). As the gliding movements occur small dilation fields (Fig. 19-10, dilation arrows at *3*) form that give rise to the arrector pili muscles. The sebaceous gland related to the hair differentiates in a small parathelial liquation field in the angle between the arrector pili muscle and the epidermis.

All late differentiations take place on the basis of the numerous metabolic fields that developed earlier. The late differentiations in turn impart new abilities and consequently new potentialities for further development.

20

DETRACTION FIELDS

CLASSICAL HUMAN ANATOMY, as well as classical comparative anatomy, was based primarily on osteology. Today, it is known that the formation of bone is not crucial for differentiations to occur. The first ossifications do not appear until the end of embryonic development in the second month when most of the more complicated differentiations are clearly distinct. From the topokinetic viewpoint there are three types of osseous tissue: 1) Bone that develops from stretched connective tissue (membrane bone); 2) bone that develops from cartilage (cartilage bone); and 3) bone that develops from already formed osseous tissue. The last type exhibits the most complicated differentiations, the Haversian system. All three types have a common developmental kinetic feature in that all ossification processes are always accompanied by an extensive hardening of the intercellular ground substance. This extracellular phenomenon is crucial to the initiation of the ossification process. Mesenchymal cell aggregations that slide along such hardened supports are pressed onto these supports. Fluid is lost from the ground substance which consequently hardens. Zones in which cell aggregations slide with friction along a hardened support are called *detraction fields* (Fig. 20-1).

Because hardening of the ground substance is an important "pre-function" for ossification it is understandable that osseous

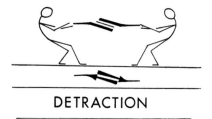

DETRACTION

Figure 20-1. Simplified demonstration of the developmental movements associated with detraction fields. The matchstick man on the left pulls a hardened plate that is adherent to a similar plate which is being pulled in the opposite direction by the man on the right. The pull on the plates gives rise to frictional forces. Similarly, mesenchymal cell aggregations in vivo slide along hardened ground substance (sliding arrows) and are variably compressed. The ground substance loses fluid and hardens. Zones in which tissue slides along a hardened support with friction are called detraction fields. Metabolic processes arise in such fields which lead to an intense squeezing out of fluid from the ground substance with subsequent hardening. Detraction fields are zones of ossification.

tissue normally appears only in late development. Early embryonic tissues have a very high water content and are not yet able to become developing bones.

The general statement that differentiation occurs only where there is spatial opportunity and an immediate kinetic (space and time) occasion is valid also for the process of ossification. For example, if the area where the frontal bone arises is examined, the following is observed. The dura mater anlage (ectomeninx) is a layer of stretched connective tissue that splits into two layers with the establishment of an ossification center on the outer layer (Fig. 20-2, *1*). The splitting is caused by the strong pull of the orbital septum in the direction of the lower face (*3*). The outer layer of the dura anlage yields to the pull. The inner layer, however, accommodates the uniform expansive growth of the arachnoid. Micrographs of a suitably sectional plane through this region show a three-angled field, the hypotenuse of which is formed by the inner layer of dura and the other two sides by the outer layer of dura. The angle between the other two sides was originally 180°, that is, they formed a continuous straight layer. In the illustrated stage (Fig. 20-2) this angle has decreased. Intercellular fluid has been released from the region which is squeezed as the angle is decreased. As a result, the ground substance became condensed

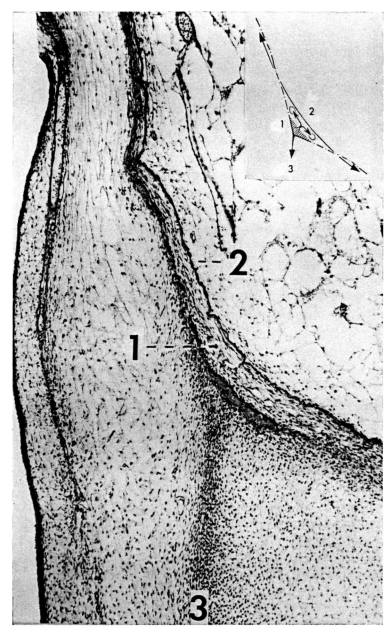

Figure 20-2. Frontal section through the face of a 27.2 mm embryo, stage 22, end of second month, 260×, showing the origin of the frontal bone. *1*, splitting area between the inner and outer layers of the dura mater anlage (ectomeninx); *2*, inner layer of dura mater anlage; *3*, orbital septum. The diagram shows the biokinetics of this region. Orbital septum (*3*) exerts a growth pull in the direction of the arrow as the brain expands; tailed arrows indicate the displacement of fluid from the ground substance which undergoes extensive hardening in the striped zone.

and hardened. In this manner a condensation center for the development of bone has been formed. On the other hand, fluid has accumulated along the hypotenuse in the interior of the triangular field. The fluid accumulation is part of the local differentiation process. A highly branched venous plexus draining the fluid is located in the area. This local differentiation process is another example of separation processes, which have been observed more than once in contrary differentiations.

The metabolic movements described above are characteristic for the origin of osseous tissue. Once hardened, the interior of the tissue in the condensed area loses the ability to grow (so-called intussusceptional growth becomes impossible in the hardened zone). The tissue forming a mantle around the small condensation center then enlarges by cell proliferation and subsequent growth. In this system the condensation is a focal ossificiation point. However, kinetically it is a new reference point for the surrounding stroma which expands in a manner that results from the growing embryonic brain. With the passage of time, the ossification center expands as divergent lines radiating from the condensation point (detraction field). Older frontal bones, which have enlarged by appositional growth in accordance with brain growth, correspondingly show generally fan-shaped structures (Fig. 20-3). For additional figures see Blechschmidt, E. and Blechschmidt, M., 1977.[11]

Upon investigating a single osseous trabecula in suitable oblique sections, one finds that its superficial cells have a stream-line arrangement (Figs. 20-4 to 20-6). Measurements of the proportional changes in the growing trabeculae in micrographs lead to the conclusion that the tissue moves against resistance along the condensation zone (*see* osteoblasts in Figs. 20-5 and 20-6). This statement is supported by two observations; the osteoblasts at the pointed "stern" of the boat-like trabecular anlage are rhombic-shaped, while those at the "bow" are always typically flattened cells (Fig. 20-5). Each osteoblast develops in accordance with its

---

[11]Blechschmidt, E. *Principles of Biodynamic Differentiation,* NIH-Symposium on Development of the Basicranium, 1977. Blechschmidt, M. *Biokinetics of the Developing Basicranium,* NIH-Symposium on Development of the Basicranium, 1977.

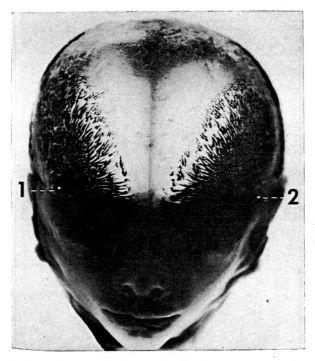

Figure 20-3. Transilluminated head of an 80 mm fetus showing the periphery of the developing frontal bones (*1, 2*). The distance between the bones increases with age. The apparently isolated osseous trabeculae are connected to the frontal bones by uncalcified trabecular segments.

kinetics. This also means that cytologically, developmental processes must also be understood in relation to position. Each cell aggregation is a unit that forms a growth functional system.

It is characteristic for osteoblasts to have their main direction tilted at a 45° angle against the surface of the osseous ground substance (Fig. 20-6). From the kinetic standpoint this arrangement is interpreted as an immediate manifestation of biomechanical shearing forces. In this regard, it is comparable to the oblique direction which muscle fibers have to their tendons (Fig. 18-6). This oblique arrangement probably results from the fact that the anlagen of the tendons, while still forming fluid precollagen, initially slide along the ends of the muscle fibers. Repeatedly an

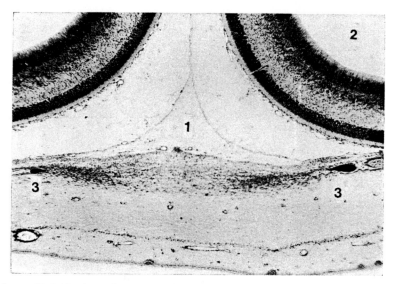

Figure 20-4 .Horizontal section through the forehead of a 50 mm fetus. 38×. The sagittal suture with the osseous trabeculae of the neighboring frontal bones has been cut obliquely. *1*, anlage of the superior sagittal sinus; *2*, cerebral hemispheres growing rapidly in surface area; *3*, osseous trabeculae of frontal bone.

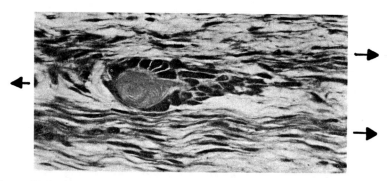

Figure 20-5. Higher magnification of the young osseous trabecula in Figure 20-4, approximately 430×. The trabecula with osteoblasts shows a streamline shape. Arrows indicate growth pull in opposite directions.

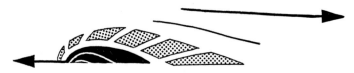

Figure 20-6. Diagram of the young osseous trabecula in Figure 20-5 showing the position and shape of the osteoblasts (stippled zones) on the layered trabecula (solid black zones).

orthogonal arrangement is often observed while frequently 45° angles are also found. This observation lends support to the concept that formative processes are immediate manifestations in uniform formative forces and are not the manifestations of single inductors.

The development of radially arranged bone is regularly modified locally. It occurs in all young osseous tissue, in so-called intramembranous bone as well as in overlying bone and cartilage bone. In other words, it occurs in all young osseous tissue which develops directly into bone from a connective tissue layer or which develops indirectly on the outside of or inside cartilage. It also occurs in all ossifications which take place after birth on previously formed osseous tissue giving rise to the trajectorially arranged trabeculae of the spongiosa and on its base, the compacta with its Haversian systems. The compacta is formed as a result of the interstices being covered over by new trabeculae.

Bones overlying cartilage characteristically develop in a field where the surrounding connective tissue is biomechanically pressed against the cartilaginous base. The nasal bone can be considered as an example (Fig. 20-7). As the cartilaginous nasal capsule broadens, the perichondrium of the nasal bridge becomes stretched. A detraction field is thereby established lateral to the cartilaginous nasal bridge underneath the perichondrium.

A special modification takes place in the distal phalanges of the fingers. As the growing cartilage in this region swells (distusion growth) in a proximodistal manner (Fig. 17-7, distal arrow), the adjoining connective tissue around the terminal end of the phalanx becomes stretched and spreads in a proximal direction (Figs. 20-8 and 17-7). This arrangement is a manifestation of the distusion function of the cartilaginous end phalanx. The osseous epiphysis of the distal phalanx appears in this area. The cells do not become flattened like those in the patellar tendon which is equally flattened against the distal end of the femur and does not slide against frictional resistance. Instead, the intercellular substance is squeezed eccentrically in an oblique direction when the septa slide on the support. The intercellular substance consequently condenses, thereby giving rise to a detraction field. The same principle is true for the metabolic fields of large and

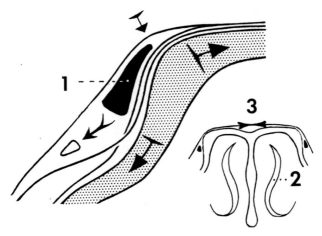

Figure 20-7. Diagram of transverse sections through the bridge of the nose of a 28 mm embryo showing the biokinetics of the formation of the nasal bones (*1*). Convergent arrows show the growth resistance of the overlying perichondrium (*3*) of the nasal capsule cartilage. *2*, nasal meatus. Divergent arrows with base lines represent the distusion growth of the nasal capsule cartilage (large stippled zone). The ground substance in zone *1* (nasal bone) hardens as fluid (tailed arrow) leaves the ossification area. Compression of the area by growth resistance of the perichondrium is shown by the uppermost arrow.

small tuberosities which are also subordinate to the rules of detraction.

On the basis of regional comparisons of developmental movements the transformation of bones can be explained under the viewpoint of developmental dynamics. For example, if the frontal bone of a fetus is strongly arched in accordance with the shape of the brain then new growth conditions arise when the cranial bones separate more and more from each other and the underlying dura flattens as a result of the increasing circumference of the brain. The external part of the young frontal bone which is initially highly vaulted is then pressed more and more against stretched connective tissue. On the other side, the internal part near the cranial cavity is detached from stretched, flattened connective tissue. Externally, between the bone and connective tissue, the movement against resistance (frictional sliding) is so impeded

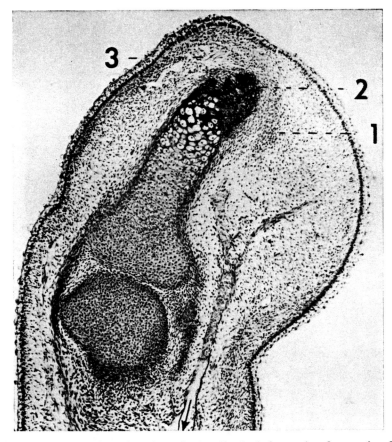

Figure 20-8. Sagittal section through the distal phalanx of a finger of a 36 mm fetus, third month, 100×, showing a detraction field at the distal end of the cartilaginous phalanx. Arrow represents the restraining function of the proper digital artery. *1*, zone of stretched tissue; *2*, zone of condensed osseous ground substance; *3*, peripheral loosened zone giving rise to veins.

that osteoclasia occurs instead of osteogenesis. The cells along the outside of the bone on the border between the fibrous stretched periosteum and the ossified tissue become deformed, flattened osteoclasts. However, the cells along the inside have the characteristic features of osteoblasts *(see* cell arrangement on concave side of the mandible, Fig. 20-9). The well-known osteocytes are typical

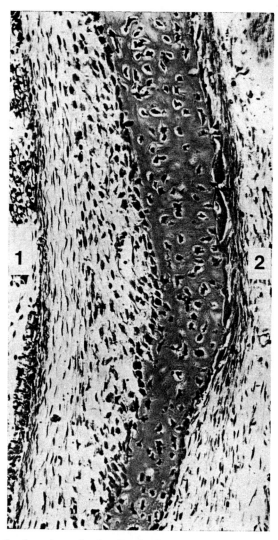

Figure 20-9. Section through the developing mandible (near the angle) of a 50 mm fetus, 210×. The situation here is similar to that of the frontal bone. Periosteum detaching from the lateral concave side of mandible contains many osteoblasts. The intussusceptional growth of the loosened periosteum causes sliding movements on the osseous support by help of the growth pull of the masseter muscle *(1)*. *2,* periosteum on the convex side of the mandible pressed closely to the bone contains many osteoclasts.

intermediate forms between osteoclasts and osteoblasts. Consequently, from the kinetic-anatomical viewpoint, one can distinguish bone-building cells (osteoblasts), bone-destroying cells (osteoclasts) and bone-preserving cells (osteocytes) in every bone undergoing transformation. This means that contrary differentiations are observed during development. All of these differentiations have metabolic factors which today are being investigated at a molecular level and, in some instances, at a submolecular level. It is implied from the kinetic-anatomical features of differentiations that the molecular and submolecular biological factors are also components of kinetic processes.

A transverse section through the tibia of an 80 mm fetus demonstrates the growth functional character of bone formation. Appositional growth with osteoblasts can be found under the periosteum (Fig. 20-10, near zone 3). Bone formation is absent in the interior of a young bone where there is a thin endosteum. As one proceeds toward the outer part of the bone there is a transition from the endosteum into the layer of osteoblasts. It becomes apparent that the mesenchyma grows out of the hard-walled bone (zone 2). Where movement with friction is rapid, e.g. on the opening of the marrow cavity in Figure 20-10, a detraction field with osteoblasts is visible. In other words, as the marrow increases in volume and expands toward the periosteum, a detraction field develops underneath the periosteum on the border of the already established bone tissue. This gives rise to subperiosteal appositional bone growth.

The formation of air sinuses in bones is the result of late differentiations that occur with very intense growth movements at bone openings (Fig. 20-11). When the head grows after birth the ossification centers (the anlagen of the left and right maxillary bones), which are near the mucosa, dislocate from each other and curve as a result of the growth pull of the zygomatic arch (simple arrows in Fig. 20-11). Consequently, beneath the lateralward dislocating bones a field with low pressure arises into which the adjoining mucosa moves quickly, laterally following the maxillary ossification center (horizontal arrows in Fig. 20-11). These developmental movements after birth result in the formation of the air sinuses.

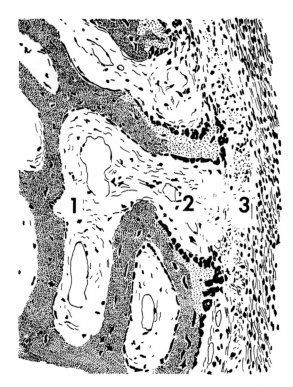

Figure 20-10. Transverse section through the tibia of an 80 mm fetus. 210×. *1*, thin endosteum which is pressed against the more rigid bony walls by the liquid-filled tissue in the chambers; *2*, outflow zone of the growing marrow (On the edges sliding movements occur in detraction fields which osteoblasts); *3*, enlarging superficial growth zone or cambium layer of the periosteum.

In conclusion, the preceding discourse has shown such harmony and so many connections between differentiation processes that it would seem illogical and unreasonable to assume that they simply share a coincidental existence. To the contrary, differentiation processes regularly follow principles that are generally valid. From the kinetic theory of ontogenetic development that has been explained it becomes clear that differentiations are developmental dynamic processes. This does not exclude other methods of examining and viewing human differentiations from being uniform in other respects, such as, with regard to their chemical pro-

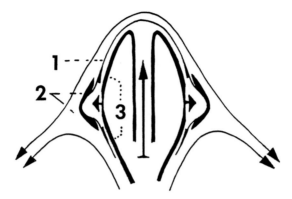

Figure 20-11. Diagram of the developmental dynamics of a paranasal (maxillary) air sinus in a newborn infant. Long arrows at periphery show growth pull of the stretched zygomatic arch which is still in the desmal state. The maxillary bone follows the pull. Growth expansion of the nasal capsule causes sliding movements on the edges of the maxillary bone. Short arrows with a base line indicate growth expansion of the mucosa. Half-headed arrows show the sliding of periosteal cells on the border of the ossification center. Large arrow shows the growth direction of the nasal septum. *1*, inner periosteal layer; *2*, maxillary bone; *3*, mucosa.

cesses or even to their psychological behavior. However, each method used does not necessarily give one an equally good synopsis of differentiations. The need for a wide survey of the connections between differentiation processes is emphasized here, because they are particularly important in today's scientific world if there is to be a clearer understanding of the voluminous data available.

GLOSSARY

Adplantation—The act of the blastocyst drawing towards and attaching to the uterine mucosa. Adplantation is followed by implantation.

Anlage—Primordium. A temporary formation that is prerequisite for the determination of later developmental processes. A quasi-blueprint for subsequent differentiations. It is not a diminutive preformation of the later differentiations and is not restricted to a particular stage of development but refers to any one of a series of stages a structure passes through during its differentiations.

Articulation loop—A tissue connection between the anlagen of antagonistic muscles. Due to this connection, the joint clefts become established.

Axial process—A part of the ectoderm which is invaginated into the interior of the entocyst disc. By its retarded growth the axial process obtains importance for the total folding of the entocyst disc.

Biodynamics—The dynamic features of development of the organism. Biodynamics are manifested particularly in submicroscopic developmental movements.

Biokinetics—The kinetic features of the development of the organism.

Biomechanics—The mechanical features of the development of the organism.

Blastocyst—The one-chambered ovum. The stage of human development that arises when intercellular liquid accumulates in the interior of the blastomeric ovum.

270

Canalization zone—Intercellular pathways which prepare for the development of blood vessels.

Contusion field—*See* Figure 15-1.

Corrosion field—*See* Figure 13.1.

Densation field—*See* Figure 14-1.

Detraction field—*See* Figure 20-1.

Development—Not only a continuous progression, but also to some extent a regression in which cell necrosis occasionally occurs, thus giving rise to new processes.

Developmental kinetics—The science of the developmental movements. They are distinguishable by the changes in position, shape and inner structure of body parts.

Developmental movements—Manifestations of spatially ordered (directed) metabolic movements which characterize the development. The position, shape and inner structure of an organ at any one stage of its differentiation are but momentary views of developmental movements which, in vivo, always occur against resistance and are therefore genuine performances in the biological and physical sense.

Development of functions—Organic differentiation is not only a development of structures but also of functional processes. The kinetics of the functions are a manifestation of the early development.

Differentiation direction—Differentiation processes start at the outside and proceed to the inside. They originate principally on the cell limiting membrane and not in the nucleus. During normal development an external stimulus is only a stimulus and not a mandate.

Dilation field—*See* Figure 18-1.

Distusion field—*See* Figure 16-1.

Dorsal entoblast chamber—A positional term for the early amniotic cavity containing the dorsal blastem or early amniotic fluid.

Ectoblast—A positional term for the outer limiting tissue of the ovum. Only where it has become particularly thick is it referred to as the trophoblast.

Embryo—The developing human being from the third to the eighth week of gestation that arises from the endocyst disc and becomes the fetus.

Endotrophe—Nutrients that arise from inside the conceptus as a result of specific metabolic processes such as liquifaction of existing cells. Compare exotrophe.

Entoblast—A positional term for all the inner epithelium of the two-chambered ovum (dorsal and ventral entoblast chambers filled with dorsal and ventral blastem fluid, respectively).

Entocyst—A positional term for the two-chambered entoblast together with its covering mesoblast.

Entocyst disc—A positional term for the disc-shaped bilaminar anlage of the embryo between the dorsal and ventral blastem fluid.

Exotrophe—Nutrients that arise outside the conceptus from perished maternal cells. Compare endotrophe.

Expansion dome—The domed cranial end of the entocyst disc that results from the expansion growth of the ectoderm with less expansion of its basement membrane (contrast impansion pit).

Fluxion—Intracellular flow in growing embryonic neurons that is an important factor in the development of the pathways.

Formative function—Pertains to an organic performance which manifests itself as a formation. All body parts, including the fluids in the body cavities, contribute to the formation of an organism and therefore have formative functions.

Gliding zone—A zone where adjacent tissue layers move in opposite directions along their substrata thereby giving origin to tissue discontinuities, e.g. synovial bursa and sheaths, joint cavities.

Hereditary factors—Genes. Prerequisites for development. How-

ever, they are only parts of metabolic fields. They are not pre-
formations in the sense of containing blueprints for later differentiations. Essentially, they are sites of application for external
differentiation forces and have only passive forming functions that
respond to external stimuli.

Impansion pit—The depressed region of the entocyst disc, that is
the result of reduced growth conditions. The ectoderm and endoderm in this region are closely compressed with little space between them for the transport of nutritive substances. Contrast
expansion dome.

Inner tissue—All tissue that is enclosed by limiting tissue during
early development. Inner tissue of the ovum is called mesoblast;
inner tissue of the entocyst disc is called mesoderm; inner tissue of
the embryo is called mesenchyma. Depending on their position,
the cells of the early inner tissue show local differences. As a
result, they exhibit dissimilarities in metabolic activity.

Limiting tissue—Tissue that is located between inner tissue and
fluid (position), becomes thicker during hindered surface growth
and thinner during increased surface growth (form), depending
on its degree of curvature, is composed of wedge-shaped cells
(structure). An extension of the word, epithelium. Limiting
tissue that is mainly composed of wedge-shaped cells is referred to
as wedge epithelium. Compare inner tissue.

Maintenance of individuality—During development, the phenomenon of an organism changes but not its intrinsic nature.
Even the ovum has an individual specificity.

Mesenchymal condensation—Dense mesenchyma. Mesenchymal
region with large numbers of closely positioned cells (high tissue
density). Superficially, near the ectoderm, it results from the intense assimilatory activity of the cells with the subsequent proliferation and compressing of each other, e.g., early dermis. Internally, away from the ectoderm it results from the intense libera-
tion of fluid intercellular substance and attraction to each other,
e.g. precartilage.

Metabolic field—A region of spatially ordered (directed) metabolic movements that is morphologically definable, e.g., retension field, contusion field, distusion field. Metabolism should not be considered only as a chemical process. A knowledge of the mechanics of metabolism is essential for a more precise evaluation of the processes involved. The brain is an example of a metabolic field. It shows directed metabolic movements which are manifested in the alignments of its fibers. The concept of fields extends from microscopic to submicroscopic anatomy.

Metabolic movements—Movements of submicroscopic particles that can be indirectly defined morphologically. Developmental movements are made up of metabolic movements that are spatially ordered. They are always components of circulatory processes.

Outside-inside differentiation—This direction of differentiation is a basic law of ontogenetic development.

Ovum—The fertilized human ovum that is either one large cell or is subdivided (cleaved) into smaller cells (blastomeres) when it is then called a blastomeric ovum. In the middle of the first week it becomes one-chambered (blastocyst). At the end of the first week it becomes two-chambered (entoblast with ventral and dorsal entoblast chamber). In the second week the human ovum is three-chambered (with yolk sac cavity, amniotic cavity and chorionic cavity).

Parathelial suction field—See Figure 19-2.

Parathelial loosening field—See Figure 19-1.

Parmeation—Metabolic movements parallel to membranes.

Permeation—Metabolic movements perpendicular through membranes.

Position, shape and inner structure—Morphological descriptions require the determination of all of these features. They are morphological features in different orders of magnitude. Position means the locational relationships; shape means the outer form; inner structure means the inner form.

Restraining function—All fibers, blood vessels and nerves in the growing organism act as restrainers and thus have forming functions in that they are specifically aligned resistances to growth.

Retension field—See Figure 17-1.

*Stemmkörperfunktion—*The biodynamic pressure effects (piston-like action) of distusion fields.

*Theory of development—*Blechschmidt's "biodynamic theory of development" states that the processes of ontogenesis always occur as directed metabolic movements in metabolic fields.

*Trajectorial structure—*A structure that shows a distribution of growth tensions so that their main directions are arranged perpendicular to each other.

*Trophoblast—*The thickened part of the ectoblast.

*Ventral entoblast chamber—*A positional term for the yolk sac cavity containing the ventral blastem or yolk sac fluid.

*Wedge epithelium—*Curved epithelium with wedge-shaped cells. Depending on the degree of curvature, the cell limiting membranes at the sides of the cells, which are always perpendicularly aligned to the basement membrane, either converge (convergent wedge epithelium) or diverge (divergent wedge epithelium) to the free surface after the epithelium becomes curved. Growth rates of convergent and divergent wedge epithelia are usually different.

CITED LITERATURE

Blechschmidt, E.: *The Stages of Human Development Before Birth.* Saunders, Philadelphia, 1961 (in text: 1961).

Blechschmidt, E.: *Die Pränatalen Organsysteme des Menschen.* Hipokrates Verlag, Stuttgart, West Germany, 1973 (in text: 1973).

Blechschmidt, E.: *The Beginning of Human Life.* Springer-Verlag, New York, 1977 (in text: 1977).

Gasser, R.F.: *Atlas of Human Embryos.* Harper and Row, Hagerstown, 1975 (in text: 1975).

INDEX

A

Adplantation, 11-12
Air sinuses
  developmental dynamics, 269
  formation, 267, 269
Alimentary canal, 132
Allantois, 60
Amnion, 15, 20, 23, 28, 69
  kinetics, 27
Amniotic cavity, 69
  movement of katabolites, 44
Amniotic fluid, 19
  origin, 19
Anlage
  definition, 4
Aorta (see Arteries)
Arachnoid (see Meninx)
Arachnoid fluid, 66
Arm
  growth grasping movement, 178
  morphokinetics, 160
Artery(ies)
  aorta, 60, 82-84, 185
    anastomoses between dorsal and
      ventral, 130
    anlage, 48, 59
    dorsal branches, 62
    metameric branches, 63-64
    restraining function, 83-84, 127, 179
    ventral, 85
  first arch, 85
  formation, 18
  high pressure in, 44
  intersegmental, 59-60
  lengthening rate, 44
  metameric, 59-60
  spinal, 185-186
Articulation loop, 206-207
Axial process, 30-40
  biodynamics, 38
  constructive importance, 38

Hensen's node, 34-37
"rolled rim" area, 34-37

B

Basal ganglia, 109-111
Basicranium, 131
  densation field, 191
Bending folds, 126
Bilateral symmetry, 47
Biogenetic law, xii
Blastocoel, 13-15, 20
  blastocyst liquid, 12
Blastocyst, 10-13
  liquid, 12
Blastomeres, 11
Blastomeric ovum, 10, 11
Blood islands, 26
Blood vessels, 80-87 (see also Arteries
  and Veins)
  restraining function, 82, 84
  topokinetics, 80-82
Body stalk
  mesenchyma, 44
Body wall, 70-77
  anlage, 40-42
  dorsal, 66-67
  growth, 157
  ventral, 66
Bone(s) (see specific bones and Ossification)
Brachial plexus, 104
Brain (see also specific parts)
  ascent, 132-134
  basal ganglia, 109-111
  centers, 104-110
  central pathways, 104-110
  cerebralization, 132, 143
  forebrain, 108
Bronchial tree, 250

C

Canalization zones, 81-82
Capsula pellucida, 5, 8
Cardialization, 143
Cartilage
    development, 202
    distusion function, 205, 238
    formation in contusion fields, 194, 202
    location, 202
    swelling growth, 203
    young cell, 202
Cell(s)
    longitudinal growth of aggregations, 39-41
    necrosis, 183-184
    reduction in volume, 183
    shape in contusion fields, 196-199
Cerebellar hemispheres, 89-90
Cerebral cortex, 108-110
    trajectorial structure, 110-111
Cerebralization, 132, 143
Chorion(ic)
    cavity, 24, 25
        nutrient absorption, 44
Choroid plexuses, 110
    mesoblast, 23, 29
    nourishment of entocyst, 43
    pole, 29
    villi, 27
Chromosomes, xi-xiii, 6
Cleavage, 7
Cloacal membrane, 185
Coelomic cavity, 61
    extraembryonic, 55, 65
    intraembryonic, 45, 65, 66
Colon
    anlage, 78-79
    dilation fields, 242-243
Contusion field(s), 30, 51, 194-200
    associated cell shapes, 196-198
    associated kinetic movements, 194-195
    biodynamics, 198
    biokinetics, 195
Corium (*see* Dermis)
Corrosion field(s), 183-186
    associated metabolic movements, 184
    examples, 185
Cranial nerve(s), 102-103

olfactory, 136
    restraining function, 136
optic, 99
positional relationships, 102
trigeminal, 112-113, 127
Cutis (*see* Skin)

D

Densation field(s), 187-193
    associated kinetic movements, 188
    biodynamic process, 192-193
    in basicranium, 191
    in nasal septum, 191-192
    in skeletal anlage, 188
    in tracheal anlage, 189-190
    significance of position, 188
Dermatome(s), 62, 231
Dermis, 170-171 (*see also* Skin)
    biokinetics, 224
Detraction field(s), 257-269 (*see also* Ossification)
    associated developmental movements, 258
Developmental movements
    general, xiii, 9
    ovum, 10
Diaphragm, 138-140
Diencephalon, 51
Differentiation(s)
    developmental dynamic, 3
    direction, xiii, 29, 35, 37, 76
    general, 6
    of cytoplasm, 55
    principles, xi, xiv
    relativity, 3
Dilation field(s), 228-243
    associated developmental movements, 229
    in colon, 242-243
    in differentiating somite, 234
    in early heart, 229-231
    in elbow, 234
    in proximal forearm, 236
    in small intestine, 240, 243
    location, 228
    relationship to distusion fields, 237-238
Distusion fields, 201-212

associated developmental movements, 201

Dorsal aorta *(see* Arteries)

Dorsal blastem fluid, 19, 28

Dorsal entoblast chamber, 28

Duct
mesonephric, 64
Wolffian, 64

Dura mater *(see* Meninx)

E

Ear
importance of cranial neuropore, 51-53

Ectoblast, 17, 18, 21, 26
growth rate, 23

Ectoderm, 15, 16
biokinetics, 75
blood supply, 76
growth rate, 42
nourishment, 43

Ectodermal ring, 72-76

Ectomeninx *(see* Meninx)

Elbow
biodynamics during development, 236
dilation fields, 236.

Embryo, early, 42
metabolic movements, 43
nourishment, 43
sandle shape, 42

Embryonic disc *(see* Entocyst disc)

Endocrine gland(s), 29
topokinetics, 84-87

Endoderm, 15, 16, 20
biokinetics, 75
growth rate, 42
nourishment, 43

Endomeninx *(see* Meninx)

Endotrophe, 25

Entoblast, 15, 17, 21
growth rate, 23

Entocyst, 15, 23, 29
nourishment, 43

Enotcyst disc, 20-29, 40
developmental movements, 32
dorsal bulges, 37, 40
ectoderm, 32
endoderm, 33
expansion dome, 30, 31, 34, 35, 36

head process, 36
impansion pit, 30, 31, 34, 35
inner tissue, 33
limited tissue, 33, 34
limiting tissue, 33, 34
mesoderm, 33

Epiphysis
of phalanges, 208
trajectorial structure, 208

Epithelium *(see also* Limiting tissue)
diathelia, 183
divergent wedge, 29

Excretory apparatus
early developmental movements, 67

Exotrophe, 17

Expansion dome, 28, 39, 30, 31, 37

Extragenetic information, xi, xiii, 9, 29, 55

Eye
importance of cranial neuropore, 51-53

F

Face, 127-136, 216-220
biokinetic movements, 191-192
kinetics, 132
lengthening, 132-134
lower lip movements, 245-247
morphogenesis, 219
supranasal sulcus, 216-218
zygomatic arch, 269

Field(s)
contusion, 194-200
corrosion, 183-186
densation, 187-193
detraction, 257-269
dilation, 228-243
distusion, 201-212
early metabolic, 5, 6, 9-179
early ovum, 10
late metabolic, 181-269
metabolic, 6
parathelial loosening, 244-256
retension, 213-227
suction, 244-245

Finger
densation fields, 196-198
developmental kinetics, 204, 223-224

distusion fields, 203-210
epiphysis, 208
main alignments of mesenchyma, 197
ossification of phalanges, 263, 265
Fluxion zones, 112
Foot
    growth architecture of heel, 226-227
Forearm
    biodynamics in proximal part during
        development, 236
    dilation fields, 236
Forebrain, 108, 127
Frontal bone, 258-262
    biokinetics, 259

G

Genes, xii
Genetic information, 55
Germ disc (*see* Entocyst disc)
Gland(s)
    adenomeres, 249-250
    biodynamics, 248-250
    endocrine, 29, 250
    formation in suction fields, 244-251,
        254
    growth direction, 249
    suprarenal, 250
    sweat, 254
Gut (*see* Intestine)

H

Hair germ, 255-256
Hand plate, 169-170
    main alignments of mesenchyma, 170
Head process, 36
Heart
    anlage, 45-48
    cardialization, 143
    descent, 140
    dilation fields, 229-231
    early, 230
    inflow path, 48
        liver angle, 139-140
        liver mass, 140
    position, 45-48
    S-shaped, 48
    X-shaped, 45
Heel

growth architecture, 226-227
Hensen's node, 34-37
Hepatization, 143
Hereditary factors, xii
Hip
    biodynamics of growth, 238
Hyoid arch, 50
Hypolingual arch, 50
Hypophysis, 85-87
    neurohypophysis, 86-87
    orohypophysis, 86-87

I

Impansion pit, 30, 31
Implantation, 12-15, 17
Inducer, 37
Induction, 37, 53
Infiltration, 25
Inner tissue, 23, 33, 183
    relationship to limiting tissues, 183
Intercellular substance function, 168
Intervertebral discs, 64, 66
Intestine (*see also* specific parts)
    biokinetics, 239-243
    colon, 241-242
        developmental kinetics, 241
    dilation fields, 239-243
    roof, 55
    small, 239-240, 242-243
        developmental kinetics, 243
Intracellular circuit
    ovum, 9

J

Joint
    anlagen, 206-207
    articulation loop, 206
    formation (*see* Articulation loop)
    interphalangeal, 206

K

Kidney, 144-155
    biokinetics, 154-155
    Bowman's capsule, 154
    capsule, 144, 151
    cortex, 144, 151
    early excretory function, 147
    glomerulus, 151-154

medulla, 144, 151
nephron, 152-154
  corrosion fields, 153-154
  trajectorial alignment of limiting membranes, 152
  topokinetics, 144

L

Ligament(s)
  formation in retension fields, 215-216
  interorbital, 216-218
  restraining function, 208
Limb(s), 156-179
  artery anlage, 179
  biokinetics of upper fold, 160
  bud, 158
  early position, 156-164
  early shape, 156-164
  early structure, 164-172
  formative function of ectoderm, 163
  growth flexion
    of anlage, 175
    of digits, 177
    of elbow, 179
  growth grasping movement of upper, 178
  growth movements, 174-180
  lower anlage, 161
  marginal ridge, 165-166, 173
  nerves, 164
  paddle-shaped, 162
  placode, 158
  plate movements, 172-178
  rays of metacarpus, 177
  serosal-neural tube angle, 157-159
  skeleton, 173-177
  topokinetics, 156
  trajectorial structure, 168-172
  upper anlage, 161, 162, 168, 172-178
Limiting membranes
  function, 168
Limiting tissue(s), 16, 22, 33, 34, 183
  hindered, 45
  relationship to inner tissue, 183
Lips
  developmental movements, 245-247
Liver, 138-140
  hepatization, 143

prerequisites for growth, 138
Longitudinal growth
  dorsal bulges of endocyst disc, 39-41
  epithelium, 39-41
Loosening field, 244
Lower extremity
  biodynamics of growth, 238
Lumbrosacral plexus
  formation, 104
Lungs, 139, 140, 142
Lymph nodes, 219
Lymph sac
  fluid congestion and retension fields, 218-220
  jugular, 218-220
Lymphatics
  formation, 18

M

Mandible
  detraction field, 265-266
Mandibular arch, 50
Marginal ridge, 165-166
  basal layer, 164
  importance for skeletalization, 173
  intermediate layer, 165
  periderm, 164
Maxillary process, 130
Meckel's cartilage, 134
Membrane(s)
  bucconasal, 185
  buccopharyngeal, 185
  cloacal, 185
  in corrosion fields, 185
  oronasal, 185
  oropharyngeal, 185
Meninx(ges)
  arachnoid, 97
  dura mater, 90, 108
    anlage, 259
    densation field in, 191
    early, 94-95
    dural girdles, 89
  ectomeninx, 66, 95, 259
  endomeninx, 110
  falx cerebri, 90
  pia mater, 91
  primitive, 94-95, 100

tentorium cerebelli, 90
Mesenchyma
  plate-like, 71-72
Mesoblast, 22, 23, 26, 29
  chorionic, 23, 29
  constructive function, 32
  covering, 23, 29
  formation, 23
  marginal, 32
  yolk sac, 24
Mesoderm, 33
  entocyst disc, 40, 44
  origin, 42
  position, 40, 44
  shape, 40, 44
  structure, 40, 44
  unsegmented, 55
Mesonephric
  duct, 64, 145, 147
  tubule, 64, 67
Metabolic field(s) (*see* Field(s))
Metabolic movements
  diathelial, 59
Metamerism, 59
Metanephrogenic diverticulum, 147
Metanephrogenic mass, 146-149
Metencephalon, 89
Mitosis
  positional dependence, 28, 29
Mouth
  early, 48
Muscle (*see also* Dilation fields)
  biodynamics of cardiac, 229
  biodynamics of smooth, 239
  location, 228
Myelination
  nerve fibers, 122-124
Myotome(s)
  formation in dilation fields, 231-234

N

Nasal bone(s)
  biokinetics, 264
  detraction field, 264
  ossification, 264
Nasal capsule, 134-136
  distusion growth, 264
Nasal pit

morphokinetics, 130
  topokinetics, 130
Nasal placode (*see* Olfactory placode)
Nasal septum, 191-192
  biokinetic movements, 192-193
  densation field, 191-192
Neck
  configuration, 141
  formation, 141
Nerve(s), 98-104 (*see also* Cranial nerves
    and Spinal nerves)
  construction, 98
  facioacoustic, 50
  shape, 98
  trigeminal, 50
Nerve fibers
  growing tips, 110-115
  growth fluxion, 119
  motor, 120-122
    biokinetics, 120-122
    developmental movements, 118
  myelination, 122-124
  peripheral glia, 122-124
  positional relationships, 115
  Ranvier's nodes, 123
  Schwann cells, 122-124
  sensory, 115-120
    biokinetics, 122
    developmental movements, 115, 118,
      119
    early innervation, 116-117
Nerve plexuses, 164
Nervous system (*see also* specific brain
    parts, Neural tube, *and* Nerve(s)
  growth rate, 94
Neural arch (*see* Vertebral arch)
Neural crest, 94-95, 100
  formation, 95-96
Neural epithelium, 92
Neural groove, 38, 39, 59
  closure, 48-51
Neural process, 66
Neural tube, 157
  ependymal layer, 92-93
  inner zone, 92
  intermediate zone, 92
  mantle layer, 92-93
  marginal layer, 91-93

outer zone, 92
position, 88-91
shape, 88-91
structure, 91-93
wall, 91
Neurocoele, 61
Neuropore
   caudal, 55, 60, 63
   cranial, 50-51
      biodynamics, 51-53
Nose, 216-220
   ossification of nasal bones, 264
   supranasal sulcus, 216-218
Notochord, 86-87
   anlage, 30-37
Notochordal process (*see* Axial process)

O

Olfactory placode, 127
   morphokinetics, 130
   topokinetics, 130
Ontogenetic law, 3
Optic sulcus, 50-53
Optic ventricle, 51
Optic vesicle, 127
Orbital septum, 259
Oronasal membrane, 185
Oropharyngeal membrane, 185
Ossification
   biokinetics, 260-262
   bone cells, 265
   bone marrow, 267
   cartilage bone, 263
   in detraction fields, 257-269
   mandible, 266
   membrane bone, 258
   tuberosities, 264
Osteoblasts, 265
Osteoclasts, 265
Osteocytes, 265
Otic placode, 50
Otic vesicle, 127
Ovum
   adplantation, 11-12
   bilaminar, 16
   blastomeric, 10-15
   capsula pellucida, 5, 8
   cleavage, 7-9

developmental movements, 10
equator zone, 18
general, xi-xiii
implantation, 12-15, 17
intracellular circuit, 9
one-cell, 5
oxygen consumption, 7, 11
poles, 18
shape, 28
shape retension, 19
three-chambered, 24
trajectorial structure, 19
two-chambered, 13-16, 22
volume, 12
zona pellucida, 5, 8

P

Palatine process(es), 134-136, 185
   in corrosion field, 185
Parathelial loosening fields, 244-256
Parathelial metabolic movements, 59
Parmeation, 25, 26
Pericardium
   descent, 140
Permeation, 25, 26
Phalanx(ges)
   anlage, 203-205
   biokinetics, 209-210
   distusion function of cartilaginous an-
      lage, 203, 205
   ossification, 263, 265
Pharyngeal arch(es), 207, 125-131
   first (mandibular), 125-126
   fourth (lower laryngeal), 125-126
   second (hyoid), 125-126
   third (upper laryngeal), 125-126
Pharyngeal groove
   first, 129
Pharyngeal pouch
   first, 127, 129
Pia mater (*see* Meninx)
Pituitary gland (*see* Hypophysis)
Placenta
   lacunae, 18
Pleural sacs, 140
Pleuropericardial cavity, 45-48
Postcardinal vein
   constructive function, 144

Potentialities
  importance of circumstances, 54
Preventral blastem fluid, 22
Primary intestinal loop, 70
Primitive pit (*see* Impansion pit)
Primordium
  definition, 4
Prosencephalon, 51
  diencephalic part, 51

R

Rathke's pouch, 85-87
  topokinetics, 86-87
Renal calices, 146
Renal pelvis, 146
Respiratory tract
  topokinetics, 142
Retension fields, 213-227
  associated developmental movements,
    214
Retinacula
  formation in retension fields, 221
Retrositus, 64, 67
Rib(s), 66
  formation, 143-144

S

Sclerotome(s), 56, 64
Segmentation, 59
  furrows, 59, 61, 63
  septum, 61, 62
  zone, 63
Serosa, 66, 76-77, 157
Skeleton
  anlage, 168, 188
    densation fields, 188, 196
  trajectorial structure, 209-212
Skin
  anlage(n)
    hairs, 254-256
    labial glands, 247-249
    papillary system, 251-252
    sebaceous glands, 255-256
    sweat glands, 254
  biokinetics, 254-255
  dermis, 170-171
  epidermis, 164-165
    basal layer, 164

intermediate layer, 165
periderm, 164, 251
stratum basale, 251
stratum intermedium, 251
retension fields, 223
Skull
  desmal, 131
Skull base (*see* Basicranium)
Small intestine
  dilation fields, 240, 243
Somatopleura, 66
Somite(s), 54-67
  biokinetics, 57-62
  capsule, 56, 60, 62
  dermatome, 62
  developmental kinetics, 234
  differentiation, 233-234
  first day of appearance, 55
  in dilation field, 234
  sclerotome, 62
  segmentation septum, 56
Spinal Cord, 93, 98
  alignment of cell membranes, 107
  centers, 104-110
  central pathways, 104-110
  retarded growth of floor plate, 96
  trajectorial arrangement, 106-107
  U-shaped fibers, 105
Spinal ganglia, 100, 102
Spinal nerve(s), 98-104
  brachial plexus formation, 104
  dorsal root formation, 95-98
  in upper limb, 179
  lumbrosacral plexus formation, 104
  ventral root formation, 95-98
Subcutis, 171-172
  kinetics in heel pad, 225
  retension fields, 223
Submesencephalic septum, 126, 128
Suction field, 244-245
  associated developmental movements,
    245
  location, 244
Suprarenal gland, 250
Surface growth, 73-79

T

Tendon(s)
  biodynamics, 235

biokinetics, 222
formation, 214-215, 235-237
Third ventricle, 51
Thoracic wall, 140
ventral, 143
Thyroid gland, 84-85
appearance, 84-85
positional relationships, 84-85
topokinetics, 84-85
Tibia, 267-268
detraction fields, 268
trajectorial structure, 211-212
Tongue
formation, 132
Topography
cell limiting membranes, 6
cytoplasm, 6
nuclear structure, 6
Trachea, 189-190
anlage, 189-190
biokinetics, 190
densation field, 189-190
Trajectorial structure
importance of, 19
Trilaminar disc, 40

U

Umbilical area, 68, 71
Ureteric tree, 250
Urinary bladder, 150

V

Vein(s)
body stalk, 44
cardinal, 101-103
dorsal intersegmental, 100-101
formation, 18
intersegmental, 60
lengthening rate, 44

low pressure, 44
metameric, 100-101
umbilical, 44
vacuolization zones, 81
Vertebral arch, 199-200
contusion field, 199
densation field, 199
retension field, 199
Vertebral column
bodies, 62, 65
intervertebral discs, 64-66
relationships, 65
Vessel formation, 18, 26, 43, 44, 59 (*see also* Artery, Lymphatics *and* Vein)
Viscera
descent, 132-133, 137-142
Visceral arches, grooves and pouches (*see* Pharyngeal arches, grooves *and* pouches)
Vitelline duct, 70

W

Wedge epithelium, 29, 39
formative function, 148-150
Wolffian duct (*see* Mesonephric duct)

Y

Yolk sac, 15, 26, 27, 69-70
absorption of nutrients, 44
endoderm, 26
function, 29
kinetics, 27
mesoblast, 24
secondary, 17
Yolk stalk, 70

Z

Zygomatic arch
formation, 131